BULIMAREXIA
THE BINGE / PURGE CYCLE

BULIMAREXIA

The Binge / Purge Cycle

MARLENE BOSKIND-WHITE, PH.D.
WILLIAM C. WHITE, JR., PH.D.

W·W·NORTON & COMPANY   New York · London

Some of the material in chapter 7, "The Treatment of Bulimarexia," appears in different form as a chapter in *Binge Eating: Theory, Research and Treatment* (eds.: R. C. Hawkins II, W. J. Fremouw, and P. F. Clement), Springer Publishing Company, New York.

Published simultaneously in Canada
by George J. McLeod Limited, Toronto.
Printed in the United States of America.

The text of this book is composed in Baskerville, with display type set in Goudy. Manufacturing by The Maple-Vail Book Manufacturing Group. Book design by A. Christopher Simon.

First Edition

Library of Congress Cataloging in Publication Data

Boskind-White, Marlene
  Bulimarexia: the binge/purge cycle.

  Includes index.
  1. Bulimarexia.   2. Women—Mental health.
I. White, William C., Jr.   II. Title.
RC552.B84W47   1983   616.85'2   82–14374

ISBN 0-393-01650-1

W. W. Norton & Company, Inc. 500 Fifth Avenue, New York, N.Y. 10110
W. W. Norton & Company Ltd. 37 Great Russell Street, London WC1B 3NU

1 2 3 4 5 6 7 8 9 0

For our daughters

DEBORAH, REBECCA, AND KIM

*May they achieve womanhood in a society
that values both mutuality and independence.*

For our sons

JON AND CLINT

*May they achieve manhood in a society where honesty,
respect, and equality for both sexes
allow them to experience the joys
of intimacy and genuine partnership.*

Contents

Acknowledgments

From conception to completion, this book took five years. Without the hundreds of bulimarexic clients who educated us during this time, it would never have happened. This is truly their book—a tribute to their trials and tribulations. From their strengths and moments of weakness, much valuable learning emerged. We are proud to have known and worked with these women and want to acknowledge their enormous talent and potential. Although the accounts they have contributed are true, in every case we have changed names and other details in order to protect their identities.

We are indebted to a number of prominent social scientists and psychotherapists whose work helped immeasurably in the formulation of our research and treatment program. Although out treatment does not espouse any one school, our thinking with regard to dynamic concepts and therapeutic style has been strongly influenced by the work of Alfred Adler, Albert Bandura, Eric Berne, Albert Ellis, William Glasser, and Fritz Perls. Additionally, Marlene's consciousness was raised and her approach to therapy with women was significantly shaped by Betty Friedan, Phyllis Chesler, and Stella Resnik.

There are others whom we thank for their contribution to the book. In addition to their painstaking review of the manuscript, Rebecca Chidester Axelrod, Jacqueline Barlow, and Drs. Sandra Bem and Hope Perry made numerous suggestions that strengthened the book in final form. Their encouragement and enthusiasm were contagious and helped us to survive frequent bouts of "writer's despair."

Our editor, Carol Houck Smith, whose task it was to help organize and present five years of clinical research, contributed significantly to the clarity and balance of our writing. We are deeply grateful for the time and energy she expended.

Sharon Greene, our superb assistant who typed several revisions of this book, also assumed major responsibility for helping us respond to the pleas for help from bulimarexics, who continue to write us daily. Without her ready support, this book would never have progressed as it did.

Much of this book was written at Gannett Health Center, Cornell University, Ithaca, New York. We are grateful to the staff of that fine institution for providing us with the necessary support and facilities.

MARLENE BOSKIND-WHITE
WILLIAM C. WHITE, JR.

BULIMAREXIA
THE BINGE / PURGE CYCLE

CHAPTER 1

The Evolution of This Book

On an early autumn evening in 1975, we attended a reception honoring a woman faculty member we had long admired for her scholarly, inquisitive mind and feminist philosophy. As we joined the reception line, we overheard several well-wishers applauding her latest work. We noticed that she turned aside these compliments with breezy disdain. Then a man ahead of us in line commented that she looked ravishing and seemed much slimmer than when he had last seen her. The woman beamed and replied, "That's the nicest compliment I have received all night."

As we drove home that evening, we were somewhat disillusioned and clearly sensitized by what we had observed. We were not yet aware of the complicated relationship between women and food or of the obsessional "fear of fatness" that underlies it. Soon, however, we began to see women who reminded us of this esteemed faculty friend—young, slim women who were obsessed with weight and who believed they were powerless in the face of food and that there just was too much of them. A patient named Suzanne provided our first personal insight into the problem. Marlene was beginning a two-year internship at Cornell University Psychological Services and was in a doctoral program in counseling. Suzanne had been randomly assigned to Marlene. During their second session, after an extended period of silence punctuated by tears, Suzanne blurted out: "I have a problem with food. I eat. I mean I eat disgusting amounts of food. You can't imagine how much I eat. I go on these binges. Then I start thinking about all those calories, and . . . and I make myself throw up. I can't stop myself. I hate myself, and I don't believe I'm telling you this."

Over the next sessions, a pattern began to emerge. Suzanne had been voted "most likely to succeed" in her small-town high school. Now at Cornell, a thousand miles from home, her high school A's had dwindled to C's, and she felt deeply guilty and ashamed that she was not living up to her parents' expectations, which were also her own: "They're spending so much money to send me here and I can't concentrate. Then I go out and spend their money on food and feel more guilt . . . and it goes on and on." In addition, though fashionably thin, Suzanne had had few dates; in fact, her social life lacked both male and female companionship.

Suzanne had spoken about her eating problems only once before—to a therapist she had seen while in high school. She had not, however, informed her therapist of the intensity, frequency, or duration of the binge / purge cycle that had been consuming so much of her energy. He had, therefore, reassured her by telling her that she was so thin she need not worry about overeating. Suzanne and her therapist spent the next six months working almost exclusively on the past, exploring issues underlying her obsession with food. Since that time, she had kept her binge-ing and purging a secret; she made sure that she was never caught in the act, so family and friends were not aware of her behavior. By the time she was nineteen, when she came to the clinic complaining of loneliness and depression, Suzanne had been binge-ing and purging three to four times a day for six years. She had read extensively about every kind of eating disorder, but had been unable to eat normally for more than a few days at a time.

Three weeks after Marlene's encounter with Suzanne, Heather, a petite, 90-pound sophomore, sought help for "heterosexual problems." She too was randomly assigned to Marlene, and she too had Suzanne's problem. "I'd rather die than be fat," she said matter-of-factly, eventually revealing that she was consuming over sixty laxatives a day after grotesque food orgies.

Within a week, Janet, a campus beauty, revealed her binge / fast cycle to Marlene, angrily blaming it on the man she loved, who had rejected her. After all-day binges, Janet starved herself for days, barely subsisting on diet pills and coffee.

After hearing these women describe such similarities in eating behavior and lifestyle, we began to question other therapists at the clinic. We learned that within the same year, each therapist had seen several patients who complained of binge-ing and purging. As a rule, these patients did not initially reveal their obsession with food. Rather, they complained of depression, unsatisfying relationships, loneliness, and anxieties of one sort or another. Clearly, as a group, they were hesitant to reveal their behavior honestly, despite the emphasis within our clinic on short-term therapy, targeting specific behaviors upon which clients wished to work, and goal contracting.

We then assigned all young women who had admitted

to a binge / purge problem to Marlene. Each woman had her own tale to tell, but the stories that emerged had a common theme: all involved inordinate dependency, the need for constant approval, shame and self-loathing, feelings of inadequacy and helplessness, and a terror of being "found out." In the early months of treatment, the women were unaware that Marlene was seeing others with the same complaint. In fact, they did not believe that other women were engaged in this behavior. Each felt that she had invented this bizarre habit, one so unspeakable that no one else would dream of doing it. Each lived in dread that her habit would be discovered and that she would be rejected because of it. One woman had begun to keep a diary in adolescence, around the time she began to binge and purge. Cryptic notes about her behavior appeared daily. "It's pretty bad today," she would write. "It" was never named or "owned" as something she chose to do.

Because we felt that isolation was at the center of the problem, we wanted to bring the women together for group therapy. At the same time, we suspected that there were probably other women at Cornell struggling with the same behavior who would benefit from a group experience. The rationale for initiating our pilot group therapy program gained further impetus when we discovered that twenty-six women had spontaneously revealed their binge / purge behavior to therapists at the clinic during the 1974 academic year. Without exception, they felt more desperate about and dominated by their binge / purge syndrome than by any other aspect of their lives. Nevertheless, they too had rarely discussed their obsession with food. Their sense of isolation, shame, and guilt apparently inhibited them in doing so. A follow-up questionnaire revealed that 96 percent had reverted to their former eating patterns within two months after treatment. Thus, although some had done well initially, they were consistently unable to sustain that progress, primarily because, as one woman put it, "I'm not strong enough when I need to be." It soon became clear that these women had lacked critical sources of support upon leaving therapy.

On January 15, 1975, we placed the following ad in our university newspaper:

> *Attention Food Bingers:* For some time now you have been locked into a cycle of gorging on food and then purging either by forced vomiting, laxatives, diuretics, or continual dieting and fasting. You often feel unable to break this cycle. A group is now being started for persons struggling with this behavior pattern. If you are interested in joining us, please call this number.

We anticipated a few inquiries, but immediately received sixty-two! All but two of the respondents were women. Over the phone, they sounded frightened and desperate. The respondents selected for group therapy were screened on the basis of the following operational definition of the problem:

1. The woman is locked into cyclical eating behavior. She first experiences an inordinate desire for food and then consumes vast quantities. Subsequently, she purges to get rid of the food via forced vomiting (often several times a day), fasting, constant dieting, laxative or diuretic abuse.

2. The woman exhibits a distorted body image. She complains of being too fat even though this perception is not shared by her therapist and significant others.

3. The woman complains of low self-esteem, and of

feelings of inadequacy, helplessness, and despair. Often isolated, she fears rejection by men, distrusts women, and expresses great shame regarding her behavior.

Of the sixty-two subjects who responded to our advertisement, thirty-five women, nineteen to twenty-six years of age, met the above criteria. All of the women, by their own admission, had been struggling with these behaviors for several years. The mean age of onset was fifteen.

In retrospect, we realized that this first advertisement drew a response from a group of women that was more severely affected than subsequent groups we have treated. Initially, the clinic was unprepared for this overwhelming response. After limiting the first group to fifteen women, we referred many women to other resources, including therapy groups at the clinic, individual therapists, and organizations such as Overeaters Anonymous. We felt compelled to treat all who wished to work with us, and, at the same time, we initiated an empirical study of three different therapy groups. These studies, which were to form the basis of Marlene's dissertation, had two major purposes: (1) to obtain a more objective description of the ways in which these women differed from a comparable group of women who did not binge and purge; and (2) to evaluate the effectiveness of group treatment.

Thus, we randomly assigned women to one-to-one therapy, group therapy, or a control group. Control group members were told that although the treatment group was filled, they could obtain one-to-one therapy, which we would provide immediately, or wait approximately three months to become part of the pilot therapy group. Most women who were randomly chosen for the control group decided to remain on the waiting list.

Treatment groups were led by Marlene and a female cotherapist. The group met weekly for eleven sessions. The present-centered, action-oriented thrust of contemporary psychology and behaviorism was emphasized in these groups because we believed that heightened awareness, assertiveness training, and contracting to work toward specific goals might help women overcome their persistent sense of isolation, shame, and helplessness. In addition, the therapists embraced a feminist treatment orientation in the belief that cultural factors facilitated the obsessional pursuit of slimness by socializing women to become passive, dependent, and accommodating and to value their bodies principally for physical attractiveness.

At the time of our initial research in 1975, the diagnostic category *Bulimia* (from the Greek and meaning "great hunger") was devoid of any reference to purging. More important, bulimia was described as a rare disorder that like anorexia (meaning to turn away from appetite), was overwhelmingly interpreted and managed within the boundaries of psychoanalytic theory. In 1955 the "Case of Laura," a slim woman who binged, was dramatized by the psychotherapist Robert Lindner in his classic book *The 50 Minute Hour*. Lindner connected Laura's oral greed with a desire to be impregnated by her father. Her "cure" necessitated an acceptance of the traditional feminine role, and Lindner's account focused on her grotesque food binges, ignoring the purging and / or starving that Laura must have engaged in in order to maintain her slim and fashionable body.

The women we were beginning to treat at Cornell found these clinical descriptions of the emaciated anorexic and the mysterious bulimic foreign and frightening and emphatically rejected psycho-sexual interpretations of their disorder. We decided to adopt a theroretical model that would more accurately describe this behavior and distinguish it from anorexia and bulimia. Thus, we coined the term *bulimarexia* and operationally defined this habitual behavior in terms of gorging, purging, and those salient dynamics that include perfectionism, obsessive concern with food and body proportions, isolationism, low self-esteem, and a strong commitment to please others, often at the individual's expense. Four years later, in 1979, independent researchers in England began to encounter a similar population of women who binged and purged. One clinician proposed the term "Bulimia Nervosa," while another chose "Dietary Chaos Syndrome" as a means of classifying the disorder.

We did not label this disorder "bulimarexia" without considering the pitfalls in doing so. The dangers of labeling a behavioral syndrome are well known. Such labeling may legitimize a behavior as a disease process so that the "victim" need assume little or no responsibility for personal actions. Being labeled mentally ill often serves to reinforce the role of the victim and the concomitant surrender of power to a healer. We were convinced that bulimarexia was a *learned behavior,* subject to the principles of learning. Since it was learned it could be unlearned. We emphasized that the lifestyle and values adhered to by the bulimarexic were maladaptive response patterns that stemmed from the process of female socialization. It was, in our view, a process consistently reinforced by the media's "ideal female."

Over a two-year period, after carefully listening and working with over one hundred bulimarexic women, we began to develop a treatment program based upon the realities these women consistently described. Rather than a desire for oral impregnation and a rejection of femininity, the belief system and lifestyle of bulimarexics overwhelmingly suggested a deeply rooted commitment to traditional feminine values. However, it was also a commitment characterized by severe conflict. The societal pressures that contributed to bulimarexia in the women we treated were identified as the very ones that cause most women in our culture to agonize over their weight.

Marlene first presented this feminist analysis of the syndrome in an essay entitled "Cinderella's Step-Sisters: A Feminist Perspective on Anorexia Nervosa and Bulimia," in the Spring 1977 volume of *Signs: Journal of Women in Culture and Society.* Another article, "The Gorging-Purging Syndrome," was published in the March 1977 issue of *Psychology Today.* This article described what we had learned from our two-year intensive study of Cornell women as well as of older women from the Ithaca community and central New York.

Despite mounting interest and inquiries from women throughout the country, we still viewed the problem as a limited phenomenon and were unprepared for the deluge of responses this article elicited. Dozens of desperate letters began arriving daily, some ten to fifteen typewritten pages long. The women poured out the pain associated with wasted years and unfulfilled dreams. They were disillusioned, frightened, and despaired that they would ever be able to control their behavior. Many who wrote were in their late twenties and thirties. Some had been binge-ing and purging for fifteen years. Others were barely in their teens: "Dr's," one began, "I am desperate and contemplating suicide because of this." One seventeen-year-old scrawled huge desperate words: "Please help me. I feel like I'm throwing up my life." All were amazed that others "did it" and were eager to know more about the problem. Most spontaneously offered to participate in our research and were eager to complete detailed questionnaires addressing a variety of familial and dynamic issues.

The *Psychology Today* article eventually drew responses from over eight hundred women ranging in age from twelve to fifty-five. Equally astonishing were letters of inquiry from over one hundred professionals, many of whom were employed in college settings. They wrote that they were seeing more and more women complaining of this problem and requested further direction regarding treatment. Bulimarexia appeared rampant not only in colleges but also in metropolitan areas and isolated rural communities. Housewives, teenagers, and professional women were thereby added to our original population.

Early group work at Cornell proved much more productive than previous one-to-one psychotherapy in that approximately half of the group members had eliminated or significantly reduced their binge-ing behavior upon six month follow up. Furthermore, the group experience was cited as critical in helping them to recognize their problem and in leading them to deal with it more actively. Nevertheless, these pilot treatment programs were not sufficient to alter critical aspects of the syndrome. In most cases, binge-ing had reinforced abnormally low self-esteem by providing an excuse for remaining isolated and not assuming day-to-day responsibilities. The increased risk taking and the changes that occurred as a result of these groups fostered new experiences, relationships, and, therefore, new problems. Follow-up studies of these women revealed one significant feature: none of the women experienced genuine intimacy in their relationships, particularly with men. Although therapy had helped to focus on developing a sense of identity independent of men, we had apparently overlooked a major goal that was spontaneously stated by most of these women—they were eager to develop or redevelop relationships with men. The all-women groups had provided few didactic or experiential opportunities for facilitating growth in this critical area; once back in the "real world," the women, soon found an opportunity to revert to binge-ing.

In the summer of 1977, after reassessing our outcome data once again, we redesigned our survey inventories and emabarked upon a group therapy program that included a male therapist. Bill, in his role as director of Cornell Psychological Services, had been actively involved with the formation of the program, but so far had remained peripheral to the direct treatment of these women. In our revised therapy program, we streamlined the eleven to twelve hours of therapy provided during a college semester into a fifteen-hour weekend marathon format. The women lived and interacted with each other for the entire weekend. One-half of our group time was devoted to individualized work with each woman within the context of the group. Three of the fifteen hours of treatment were conducted without Bill in order to maintain our emphasis on a feminist philosophy designed to facilitate the enhancement of a more androgynous identity. Bill's absence during these crucial hours also served to heighten a sense of honesty, risk taking, and camaradarie because it was much easier to talk about issues related to sexuality within an all-women group. Bill was, however, actively involved in the treatment process throughout the remaining twelve hours of therapy. In addition to providing many opportunities to observe important male / female transactions, group members were also able to interact directly with Bill, who served as surrogate father, boyfriend, and boss in role plays with women who had unfinished business. Role playing and comparable interactions provided the opportunity for women to clarify their problems with men in concrete ways, thereby helping them to acknowledge their part in relinquishing their power and perpetuating unsatisfying relationships with men. Thus, our original feminist perspective was now enhanced both by the presence of a male therapist and by the relationship training inherent in our male / female therapy team. Furthermore, the presence of a male therapist served to stimulate inquiries from fathers, husbands, brothers, and other male figures close to the lives of women in treatment. Many men were confused and angered by behavior that they were unwittingly reinforcing and consistently reached out to discuss their coping strategies with Bill. Most of them also indicated that it would have made them uncomfortable or that they would have been unwilling to express themselves in such a way to a woman therapist. From these men we received valuable insight, albeit from a different perspective, into the lives of women suffering from this secret disorder.

In August 1977 we initiated this male / female group treatment program with fourteen women who had responded to the *Psychology Today* article. Ranging in age from eighteen to forty-five, all of these women had been binge eating and purging for at least four years. Most binged daily, at least twice, and were purging one or more times during an eight-hour interval. In every case, bulimarexia was the primary maladaptive behavioral pattern. None of the women were clinically underweight or in need of medical management at the time of treatment. A letter from a physician attesting to their height, weight, and general medical condition was an admission requirement. Since this was a pilot study, we administered the California Psychological Inventory (CPI), a body cathexis test, and our survey inventory prior to the initiation of therapy, immediately after the group finished, and one year later. This time our results were more favorable, particularly with regard to eliminating or attenuating the binge-ing behavior. Furthermore, attitude changes were noted and were accompanied by a more active, ambitious, and versatile role orientation. The one-year follow-up revealed that group participants had broadened their outlook and interests as measured by the CPI and no longer loathed their bodies, as indicated by a significant increase in their body cathexis scores.

Feedback from questionnaires was especially valuable. For example, the women reported that they felt that the group size was too large. We agreed and gradually limited it in subsequent workshops, finally realizing that eight to ten women was an appropriate number. Because of other suggestions, we discarded certain techniques that the women believed were ineffectual or detrimental. One of these involved keeping a diary of daily food intake. The women felt this merely gave them permission to obsess about food during valuable group time. They believed the group was most productive when it focused on other aspects of their lives. They were tired of talking about food!

The apparent success of this first group program encouraged us to offer others. We also began to open our workshops to professionals as a teaching forum for sharing our insights and techniques. In this way, we have been able to extend our treatment to more and more women in need of help.

In September 1979 *Glamour* magazine published an article based upon interviews with us and with former clients who had agreed to share their experiences. The response to this article was so overwhelming that *Glamour* devoted its December 1979 editorial to a discussion of the enormous response that it had received. The editorial staff was staggered by the number of women who wrote, but, more importantly, it was shocked by the desperate, often hopeless message so consistently expressed:

> In September of this year, we published the article, *"Full Stomachs and Empty Lives"*, about bulimarexia, a little publicized destructive behavior pattern. . . . The reaction to this article has been startling and thought provoking—unlike any in our publishing experience—not only in the volume of mail but also in the desperate tone of many of the letters. One women described bulimarexia as "the helpless anguish, the sheer hell, in which I am drowning." "I'm not quite sure how much longer I can go on like this," wrote another, and a third woman said fatalistically "Although suicide seemed far away, nonetheless it was ultimately the only viable solution. . . ."

The *Glamour* editorial board was especially disturbed by the secrecy and shame that intensified feelings of aloneness and despair:

> Bulimarexia had been a problem for a long time, but readers who wrote us had shared it with no one. They paid the emotional toll, sometimes for years, thinking somehow that this life was all they deserved. . . . Women still hide their private terrors from the world and even from those closest to them.

Over and over again the letters said, "you mean I
am not alone?" "It hit me so hard I'm sitting here
shaking my head, I really thought I was the only
one in the world with that problem." "It is my big
dark secret of which I am terribly ashamed. . . ."

In May 1980 an article on bulimarexia by Marie Brenner appeared in *Savvy: The Magazine for Executive Women.*
Professional women from all walks of life—lawyers, physicians, dancers, athletes, psychologists, and business
women—wrote to us and revealed that they were consumed by the same shame, isolation, and despair. They too
were bulimarexics! Other articles about our work with
bulimarexic women soon followed. Feature articles in
Ladies' Home Journal and *Seventeen* brought forth another
flood of responses. Alarmed and disheartened by the
hundreds of letters from preteens, we began to concentrate on the preventive aspects of this disorder, with particular regard to students in high schools and universities.
These outreach activities have been encouraging in that a
significant number of men are attending our lectures and
asking for advice about how best to deal with girlfriends
and other loved ones struggling with the syndrome. Equally
rewarding has been our consulting work with mental health
practitioners within these institutions who are eager to learn
more effective treatment and preventive techniques.

We also act as consultants to private and public high
schools and have enjoyed regular speaking engagements
on "Health Awareness Day" and other such occasions. Such
opportunities help to fortify young women with the skills
they need to deal with the precursors of bulimarexia. We
expect to continue this kind of outreach activity in the
future as an adjunct to our applied research and work-

shops, now being offered on a monthly basis at a variety of settings throughout the country.

This book was written for bulimarexic women, all of whom long to live fully but are paralyzed by shame, insecurity, and fear of rejection. Their escape from their self-imposed pain involves relinquishing control; eventually, perhaps the damage can be averted before it manifests itself. This book is also written for the myriad young women who are not yet bulimarexic but who have the foresight to recognize their vulnerability to problems with food.

We have attempted to address the concerns of families and friends directly involved with bulimarexic and prebulimarexic women, for their support—appropriately rendered—is necessary.

Finally, it is our hope that professional therapists will profit from our errors and insights and will find within these pages suggestions that will enhance their clinical skills so that they can aid those in need of intervention.

We have researched and treated over two thousand women since Suzanne first struggled with her confession, and although we have no idea how many more women are secretly engaged in this pernicious behavior, we are convinced the number is staggering. Although treatment has been arduous, the rewards have been significant. Bulimarexic women are, in general, bright, talented, and capable. Their prognosis, in our experience, is good primarily because of their strengths and because of the fact that bulimarexia has just begun to receive serious attention from the professional community. It is our hope that this book will further heighten awareness and will help illuminate the way to more concrete means of curtailing and eliminating this destructive habit.

CHAPTER 2

The Binge / Purge Cycle

THIN IS NEVER THIN ENOUGH

Nicole awakes in her cold dark room and already wishes it was time to go back to bed. She dreads the thought of going through this day, which will be like so many others in her recent past. She asks herself the question every morning: "Will I be able to make it through the day without being totally obsessed by thoughts of food, or will I blow it again and spend the day binge-ing?" She tells herself that today she will begin a new life, today she will start to live like a normal human being. However, she is not at all convinced that the choice is hers.

She feels fat and wants to lose weight, so she decides to start a new diet: "This time it'll be for real! I know I'll feel good about myself if I'm thinner. I want to start my exercises again because I want to make my body more attractive."

Nicole plans her breakfast, but decides not to eat until she has worked out for a half-hour or so. She tries not to think about food since she is not really hungry. She feels anxiety about the day ahead of her. "It's this tension," she rationalizes. That is what is making her want to eat.

Nichole showers and dresses and plans her schedule for the day—classes, studying, and meals. She plans this schedule in great detail, listing where she will be at every minute and what she will eat at every meal. She does not want to leave blocks of time when she might feel tempted to binge.

"It's time to exercise, but I don't really want to; I feel lazy. Why do I always feel so lazy? What happened to the will power I used to have?"

Gradually, Nicole feels the binge-ing signal coming on. Halfheartedly she tries to fight it, remembering the promises she made to herself about changing. She also knows how she is going to feel at the end of the day if she spends it binge-ing. Ultimately, Nicole decides to give into her urges because, for the moment, she would rather eat.

Since Nicole is not going to exercise, because she wants to eat, she decides that she might as well eat some "good" food. She makes a poached egg and toast and brews a cup of coffee, all of which goes down in about thirty seconds. She knows this is the beginning of several hours of craziness!

After rummaging through the cupboards, Nicole realizes that she does not have any binge food. It is cold and snowy outside and she has to be at school fairly soon, but she bundles up and runs down the street. First she stops at the bakery for a bagful of sweets—cookies and doughnuts. While munching on these, she stops and buys a few bagels. Then a quick run to the grocery store for granola and milk. At the last minute, Nicole adds several candy bars. By the time she is finished, she has spent over fifteen dollars.

Nicole can hardly believe that she is going to put all of

this food, this junk, into her body; even so, her adrenaline is flowing and all she wants to do is eat, think about eating, and anticipate getting it over with. She winces at the thought of how many pounds all of this food represents, but knows she will throw it up afterward. There is no need to worry.

At home Nicole makes herself a few bowls of cereal and milk, which she gobbles down with some of the bagels smothered with butter, cream cheese, and jelly (not to mention the goodies from the bakery and the candy bars which she is still working on). She drowns all of this with huge cups of hot coffee and milk, which help speed up the process even more. All this has taken no longer than forty-five minutes, and Nichole feels as though she has been moving at ninety miles an hour.

Nicole dreads reaching this stage, where she is so full that she absolutely has to stop eating. She will throw up, which she feels she has to do but which repels her. At this point, she has to acknowledge that she's been binge-ing. She wishes she were dreaming, but knows all too well that this is real. The thought of actually digesting all of those calories, all of that junk, terrifies her.

In her bathroom, Nicole ties her hair back, turns on the shower (so none of the neighbors can hear her), drinks a big glass of water, and proceeds to force herself to vomit. She feels sick, ashamed, and incredulous that she is really doing this. Yet she feels trapped—she does not know how to break out of this pattern. As her stomach empties, she steps on and off the scale to make sure she has not gained any weight.

Nicole knows she needs help, but she wants someone else to make it all go away. As she crashes on her bed to recuperate, her head is spinning. "I'll never do this again," she vows. "Starting tomorrow, I'm going to change. I'll go on a fast for a week and then I'll feel better."

Unfortunately, deep inside, Nicole does not believe any of this. She knows this will not be the last time. Reluctantly, she leaves for school, late and unwilling to face the work and responsibilities that lie ahead. She almost feels as though she could eat again to avoid going to school. She wonders how many hours it will be until she starts her next binge, and she wishes she had never gotten out of bed this morning.

Nicole has been a binger for five years. She started binge-ing once a week and moved to several times a day after the first year. There were very few days when she did not binge. If she refrained, it was only because of "white knuckling it" (as she put it), which she could hardly main-tain for more than a day.

The binge-ing started when Nicole arrived on campus as a freshman. She gained fifteen pounds and felt alone and unable to maintain a diet. Nicole added to her isola-tion by choosing to live in a single room. Her binges increased in frequency and duration in her junior year, when she became engaged to a medical student and moved in with him. It was Allen who jokingly suggested one night that she force herself to vomit after one of her typical "poor me" dialogues about how much she had eaten and how awful she looked. Nicole's misery and shame increased as she grew thinner and more dependent on purging to off-set her binges. Allen and Nicole lived together for one year before Nicole fled the relationship for the "safety" of her family. However, since she had traded one form of depen-dency for another and was doing little more than "hanging out" at her family's home, she continued to binge and vomit. At the urging of her family, she began intensive psychotherapy, but after six months of dealing exclusively with the past, Nicole felt more hopeless and locked into the behavior than ever.

Nicole suffers from bulimarexia, a cyclical eating disorder that has reached epidemic proportions in our culture. The details of a typical day in Nicole's life are not pleasant to read about—and certainly are not pleasant to live through. Her day may differ in certain aspects from that of other bulimarexic women, but her behavior and her ways of coping with stress will be all too familiar to the thousands of women who alternately binge and then purge by self-induced vomiting, the abuse of laxatives and diuretics, or severe fasting.

Bulimarexia can affect women at any age, from the teens well into middle age. However, white middle-class adolescents and women in their twenties with a strong orientation toward academic achievement and a traditional lifestyle, including marriage, are most vulnerable. Many are highly intelligent, attractive in appearance, and capable of handling successful careers. Yet traditionally they have abnormally low self-esteem, a desire for perfection, a sense of loneliness and isolation, and an obsession with food as it relates to body weight. Some of these women feel as though they have split into two people. One is the competent woman the outside world sees; the other is the driven, out-of-control woman who will cheat, steal, or lie to satisfy her urge to binge.

In time, as the behavior increases in intensity, these women arrive at the irrational conclusion that the bulimarexic part of their personality is the "real" woman, thereby negating and undermining any successes they may experience in other aspects of their lives.

In some ways, there are similarities with anorexia nervosa, the self-starvation syndrome: the lack of self-esteem, the paralyzing sense of ineffectiveness, the distorted body image, the obsessive concern with food. Both anorexics and bulimarexics are likely to have been brought up in middle-class, upwardly mobile families, where mothers are characterized as overinvolved in their daughters' lives and fathers are preoccupied with work outside the home. For the most part, both anorexics and bulimarexics were "good children," eager to comply and achieve in order to elicit the love and approval of others.

We have, however, noted significant differences between these two groups of women. Biochemical changes that result from sustained self-starvation typically bond physiological abnormalities with psychological deficits in the anorexic. The apathy and irritability that contribute to the anorexic's unyielding stance in therapy are not as prominent among bulimarexics. Anorexics are generally younger, far less socially competent, and much more isolated from and dependent upon the family than bulimarexics. While both are obsessed with food, for anorexics eating rampages are likely to be infrequent occurrences. In sudden fits of hunger, anorexic women may binge and purge in solitude, but this is the exception rather than the rule. In fact, the anorexic is near starvation much of the time.

In contrast, the binge and purge becomes a ritual in the lives of bulimarexic women. In moments of stress, they turn *toward* food, not *away* from it. When they are able to control their behavior, they often eat highly nutritious meals in an effort to repair the harm they have done to their bodies. And, for the most part, they are able to function in social and work contexts, though not without difficulty.

Their health may certainly be affected, but their very lives are not necessarily in danger, as is often the case with anorexics. Ultimately, we have come to view this syndrome as related to anorexia yet distinct from it.

Many women teeter on the brink of anorexia or bulimarexia during adolescence. This is the time when girls become acutely aware of other girls who seem more successful and attractive than themselves. As a result, they feel inadequate or self-conscious by comparison. In searching for "magical cures" for their existential crises, both groups—preanorexics and prebulimarexics—focus on *The Diet* as their ticket to success and happiness. What happens after this first diet is crucial and critical. Their ability to resolve the frequently unfulfilled expectations about weight loss is often dependent on support from family as well as on the life experience the young women already possess. The more isolated and locked into family they are, the greater the chance they will "choose" anorexia. Anorexia represents a pathetic attempt to assert control over their lives and also over the lives of others. Women who veer toward bulimarexia are more tenacious. They do not have to "show" their pain to the extreme evidenced in anorexia. However, their passivity and desperation and their attempts to maintain control are a matter of degree; they are, in effect, stronger carbon copies of their younger, anorexic sisters.

The widespread incidence of bulimarexia has gone unrecognized until fairly recently because binge-ing and purging is in essence secret behavior. These women dread the possibility that their "disgusting" habit will be revealed, and few will tell the whole story to their doctors, therapists, or families. Even when they do, professionals and well-intentioned loved ones are often unable to provide the necessary help. Many more women, unable to confess the full truth, fall back on vague hints that are typically misread. "I told my sister and mother a partial truth about throwing up sometimes after I ate, which they interpreted as nervousness," one woman said. "I was too ashamed to tell the whole truth." When they seek out professionals, too little information is forthcoming to elicit further examination or questioning. Then, too, in our society it is assumed that women are concerned about weight and vigilant about weight control. Thus, whatever halting statements bulimarexics may make are likely to be interpreted as bids for attention or attempts to elicit flattery, rather than as cries for help. The following statement is significant:

"I never mentioned this well-kept secret to my psychiatrist, except to state that I might have a problem with compulsive eating. As I was sitting in his office in my size five dress, I'm sure he thought I was confusing an extra cookie with compulsive eating. Little did he know how adept I am at consuming a couple of family-sized packages of cookies, followed by a box of crackers, followed by three breakfast bars, followed by fifteen Ex-lax! This is just one of many eating incidents in a day."

Another woman said: "I told my doctor, sorta, but just couldn't get it all out, so he thinks I'm over it. It's too degrading and embarrassing to tell anyone about."

Obviously, bulimarexia is much more serious than an extra cookie now and then. These women must learn to be honest and to reach out for support and help in breaking the vicious cycle. This means a willingness to give up their characteristic circular thinking, a way of thought that was well demonstrated by a woman who said, "I want to be helped, but I also want to be skinny. I'd rather be skinny and have this problem than be fat and not have it."

Although bulimarexics are generally slim by any standard, they invariably *feel* fat. They appear to regard their bodies far more critically than so-called "normal women" or women with other types of emotional problems regard theirs. They are perfectionists. Thin is never thin enough. Their body proportions are *never* right. Their breasts are too small, thighs too big, and so forth.

Laura states: "I'm too heavy chested—34C is not exactly my idea of being comfortable. I feel like a freak."

Sally, who is 4'10" and weighs 110 pounds, says: "I wish my body was petite and tiny. I hate my fat legs! I wish the fat could be wished away."

Jennifer, who is 128 pounds and 5'6", feels "very unattractive if I'm over the weight I desire, even by one pound."

Marie has a petite 5'4" frame that carries all of 108 pounds. She says, "I feel like I'm too heavy now"; and Karen, at 5'8" and 117 reveals, "I love my body when it's thin. I feel hideous and fat when I'm slightly over what feels thin. My self-image is tied up with my physical beauty. I depend on people thinking I'm pretty, and if they don't, I feel crushed."

These subjective comments parallel our clinical impressions and those of many therapists with whom we have worked. In our initial work with bulimarexic college coeds, we were interested in determining the extent of their problems with distorted body image. After a search of the literature, we found a brief, straightforward, instrument, developed by Secord and Jourard, called the body cathexis test. Women are asked to rate their feelings about different parts of their body. In order to evaluate the bulimarexic, we added a few questions specifically related to the female self-image (i.e., we elicited their impressions about breasts, thighs, and being a woman). Application of this test to bulimarexic and control subjects in our early research revealed that bulimarexics loathed their bodies to a much greater extent than did women who were suffering from non-food-related problems. These findings have continued to emerge and suggest that this modified test may be a valuable diagnostic tool in helping to "discover" the elusive, bulimarexic women.

Paradoxically, our data, gleaned from the body cathexis test, also suggest that bulimarexics are quite satisfied with their gender—they very much enjoy being women. These findings cast serious doubt on the traditional "rejection of femininity" hypothesis regarding anorexia / bulimarexia in women.

In addition to feeling revulsion about their own bodies, bulimarexic women are constantly comparing their bodies—and their lives in general—to those of other women—and almost always unfavorably, with further loss of self-esteem. One gymnast who wrote to us expresses this view: "It was inexplicably painful for me just to watch in the gym. I tried to figure out who was better than me, who wasn't so good, who was fatter, and who was thinner. They were doing a complicated exercise while I agonized over the fact that I had just 'pigged out' and I couldn't attempt the movement, even if I wanted to. Feeling absolutely inadequate to do anything about myself, I would run from the gym in tears."

Such striving for perfection only helps to perpetuate feelings of despair and emptiness. On the whole, these women are articulate, bright, and talented, with a potential for creative activity. Many write, paint, dance, or act. However, for most bulimarexics these are activities of the past, activities they once enjoyed but gave up around the time they began to binge. Their conversation is peppered with such phrases as "I used to" or "Once I liked to . . ." In the present, they seem to use their memory of enjoyable activities to *intensify* their problems, so that a low–frustration tolerance coupled with unrealistic expectations practically insure failure.

More disturbing, perhaps, is that the lives of bulimarexics are devoid of fun, humor, and genuine self-pleasure. The ability and desire to participate in life joyfully have been left behind; talents and interests that once flourished have been abandoned. Psychologist Eric Berne has said that the road to freedom is through laughter. The ability to laugh also reflects insight into the absurdity of one's irrational beliefs. Humor is often a first therapeutic step toward healing. Bulimarexics, however, are somber and intense. They view life as tragic and hopeless, and their pessimistic philosophy often serves to keep more energetic and positive individuals at a distance. A majority have lost sight of or, in some cases, never discovered the child within—that crazy, fun-loving, exuberant part that permits us to reward ourselves for all we have accomplished. When we lose sight of this, our lives become dreary and meaningless. Bulimarexics typically evidence this loss of perspective.

Recently, we saw a decorative pillow that carried a message relevant to the bulimarexic's distorted sense of self: "I may not be totally perfect, but parts of me are excellent." Unfortunately, this concept is foreign to the bulimarexic who has an "ideal weight" in mind. This magic figure is definitely on the thin side, but is not clinically unhealthy as in anorexia. Those who force vomit seem to have an easier time maintaining their ideal weight than those who offset binges by fasting and dieting over longer periods of time. They weigh themselves so frequently that they can detect minute changes and act on them immediately. On the other hand, weight fluctuations in women who fast and diet after binge-ing are typically more dramatic, often ranging from 20 to 25 pounds. One thirty-six-year-old woman writes: "I binge three or four months at a time and have since junior high school. I eat everything in sight. During my binges, my weight goes up to 150 or 180. My best weight is 115 and I'm 5'6" tall. Now I'm in my 'fat phase' and I'm a physical wreck. I feel tired and unsocial. I dread being seen!"

Another woman discusses her severe cycles of weight gain / weight loss: "I've been living with this syndrome for five years. I am now twenty-years-old. My life is a perpetual diet, along with insatiable binges! I've lost 100 pounds in eighteen months. I've had many relationships and when they end I inevitably feast."

It is often difficult if not impossible to relegate women to one diagnostic category or another. Some bulimarexic women would be classified as obese during their "fat" phases. In addition, ten to twelve percent of the bulimarexic women we have treated report having been diagnosed as anorexic earlier in their lives. Several were hospitalized in order to bring their weight to medically acceptable levels. Furthermore, recent studies of women's attitudes toward food indicate that more and more so-called "normal" women are evidencing anorexic-like symptoms. This suggests that women without personality abnormalities are being pressured by unrealistic cultural standards regarding slimness. Many seem to be adopting behavior patterns quite similar to those of anorexic and bulimarexic women.

In bulimarexia one behavior elicits and sustains another.

The "bulimarexic motto" might be: "I eat to purge and I purge to eat." The disorder rarely begins as a full-blown cycle. In fact, most bulimarexics go through a phase where they are dieting, and perhaps vomiting occasionally, but they are still in control. In other words, the binge and purge episodes represent interruptions in an otherwise normal life. This early stage is short-lived and seems to end primarily because the women believe they have discovered the miracle of weight control through purging. In an overwhelming number of women, this destructive insight occurred during adolescence or early adulthood. The following two comments are typical:

"My earliest memories of the binge-ing pattern that was to be with me for the next twelve years began in adolescence. At about the age of fourteen, my best friend and I began to center our lives around visits to the neighborhood store for food, devouring packaged cakes and chocolate sundaes! If we had no money, anything we could find in her refrigerator would do. Needless to say, I began to gain weight and became quite chubby. At the end of tenth grade, I decided to lose ten pounds in order to become a cheerleader. That was the year I had my first boyfriend and was ecstatic. I was relying heavily on fasting to stay slim, which I found unbearable. In school we read about the Roman vomitoriums and I was intrigued. At first, I didn't employ this wondrous method very often but soon I reached the point where no matter what I put into my stomach, I had my fingers down my throat shortly thereafter."

"I began binge-ing and starving at age fifteen after losing fifteen pounds on a diet. This went on for a year after I became tired of starving, and I gained thirty pounds.

Having no success with dieting because I wouldn't stick to it, I began to take laxatives on occasion (one to three times per week). I then began to binge and vomit, which has been going on daily for the last two and a half years."

Forced vomiting is the most dramatic and immediate method of purging. It also appears to be the most common, perhaps because it seems to be the easiest and most efficient form of weight control. Needless to say, it may also be the most self-destructive. The issue of immediacy is probably central, because women often say that they can throw up before the calories have a chance to take effect. Vomiting also provides instant relief for their painfully overstuffed bellies.

Bulimarexics often refer to "learning" to throw up. In other words, they learn about it as a method of controlling weight. In the beginning, they seem to think it is a great new discovery. The following story illustrates this:

"In my sophomore year of high school, I learned to put my fingers down my throat to make myself throw up. I had stopped eating normal meals and would very often fast for days at a time. That Thanksgiving I had just eaten too much and I felt I was going to be sick. I was in the bathroom with my sister and cousin, and one of them said, 'Well, if it's going to come up, why don't you stick your fingers down your throat and help it up.' No sooner said than done. I felt thin again immediately and thought 'this is great! I just ate the most delicious, fattening dinner and I won't gain any weight.'"

The length of a binge depends primarily upon the method of purging. For those who purge via fasting, the entire binge / purge cycle may last a few days or extend to several months. One woman binged every day or so, then gave up eating altogether for at least twenty-four hours, sometimes forty-eight. Another had a cycle of binge-ing for one day, then dieting strenuously for the next few days. This meant skipping breakfast, having plain yogurt for lunch, and eating hard-boiled eggs and a vegetable for dinner. ("I chew gum when I feel like snacking. If I want to lose weight quickly, I limit myself to two hard-boiled eggs a day.") Still another, after periods of binge-ing, would go on a series of drastic diets, the most serious of which was a "meat" diet. "All that I ate for eleven weeks was six ounces of meat a day and diet soda; I lost thirty-five pounds and gained it back in two months, for I immediately began binge-ing again." For those who purge by forced vomiting or laxative abuse, the cycle is generally complete within an hour or two.

Other women learn about purging methods from friends. The young woman who learned about the Roman vomitoriums and was "intrigued" has already been mentioned. The technique was introduced to another adolescent by a veteran camper at a camp for overweight young adults; this person put it quite literally when she commented, "I found it a great way to have my cake and eat it, too." Still another read an article about gymnasts that mentioned the method. And there is Nicole, whose boyfriend jokingly suggested that she vomit after she complained one night about "pigging out."

Bulimarexics are suggestible women. It is unfortunate that a chance remark from family or even from a physician (one woman heard a doctor talk about "skinny girls who threw up") can lead to a syndrome that approaches addiction. The fact that bulimarexia is rampant in this country, especially on college campuses, has led some people to wonder whether or not it is contagious, in the manner of a disease. As we point out several times in this book, the *syndrome* itself is not contagious. It is a learned behavior. What is contagious is the passing along of the purge and the reliance upon it as a magic solution to weight control.

In addition to forced vomiting, other methods of purging are commonly utilized. Laxative abuse is quite frequent, as are diuretic and emetic abuse, fasting, and enemas. The women are likely to exercise compulsively, swimming many laps, running many miles, working out with barbells and weights. Some women combine different methods of exercise as well as experimenting with bizarre diets. A small percentage of women we have treated spend hours chewing food and spitting it out.

In order to facilitate vomiting, many bulimarexics rely on Q-tips and similar initiators because they prove more effective and less "disgusting" than fingers. They soon learn that drinking copious amounts of fluids facilitates vomiting. Some maintain that certain foods, such as chocolate, are useful in initiating diarrhea. As time goes by, with practice, most of them find that vomiting occurs spontaneously each time they eat. By this time, of course, their bodies have suffered grievously, and medical attention is necessary.

The actual length of time women spend binge-ing and purging can be misleading and irrelevant. They spend far more time in obsessive rumination about food, either attempting to stave off a binge or actually preparing for one. Many of these women appear to love to cook, which leads relatives and friends to overlook other aspects of their obsession. "I collect recipes," one woman wrote us. "I've sent away for every recipe booklet I could find, and my prized possessions are booklets with pictures of gooey, rich desserts. I especially like to torture myself by looking at these pictures while dieting, and I make lists of all the foods I'll eat when my diet is over. I tell my family and friends, several times a day, about the pizza I'm going to have when I get off this diet."

Other women enjoy planning elaborate dinners or large cocktail parties with "fifty different types of hors d'oeuvres." They constantly pore over cookbooks and are often praised as excellent hostesses. When the obsession with food leads to hoarding—as it frequently does—the torture becomes even more exquisite and the anxiety that results is extreme: "I feel obligated to eat what I've already hoarded, because I don't want to waste what I've bought." Another woman admitted: "I feel extremely nervous when I've hoarded so much food that I no longer have a place to hide it. When I have guests, I lock all cabinets, and if they should look into the refrigerator, I tell them a neighbor's fridge is being repaired and she's keeping all the food in mine."

Bulimarexics typically binge on high-calorie junk foods, the kind of food that may have been forbidden in childhood. Their selection of food may reflect defiance. Flavor and taste do not seem to be important, with sweets and fried foods, such as french fries, predominating. As time goes on, most become less and less discriminating about what they eat. "The foods are uglier and uglier, like globs of fried flour, oil, and sugar." Caloric intake per binge can range from one thousand to twenty thousand calories.

Obviously the single most important precondition to binge-ing is being alone, (although some women do report having a few cronies engaged in the same behavior). If the bulimarexic can count on being alone at night, she is more apt to binge at night. However, women caught up in this cycle are ingenious at finding places and times when they can be alone—at home, at work, and even in restaurants. At college, they may eat normal meals with roommates in communal dining places, but still find ways to slip food to their rooms afterward: "I think I'll get more pleasure out of it in my room. If I hear someone coming, I hide the food." Many women admit that if they were constantly supervised, they probably would not binge.

It is not surprising that bulimarexics have few friends— so much of their time is spent in supporting their habit and in keeping others from knowing about it. Some refuse to answer the telephone or the doorbell while under the influence of their "fat attacks." Others are simply too worn out from binge-ing to accept invitations or are afraid they will not be able to keep the date when the time comes. "If I was binge-ing and someone knocked on my door, I wouldn't answer. I'd tell people I'd be there and never show up." The following insightful statement sums it up: "Friends, that was a major problem. I knew a lot of people, but was alienating them because I couldn't be around them with the cycle I was in. There were all those people who were there for me to do things with if I was willing to say, 'Hey, do you want to come over?' I was scared to do it . . . to develop close friends."

A few bulimarexic women are drawn into relationships with other lonely and unhappy women. This often serves to reinforce their weaknesses rather than to enhance their strengths. Jan would binge with a friend at college: "I can remember one night, a low point in my life . . . we found every nickel we could and ran to the candy machine. There was only one kind of candy left, a peanut bar which we both disliked. Yet we pumped coins into that machine, on full stomachs, eating one peanut bar after another while crying, 'Why are we doing this?' "

Despite the enormous amount of time and energy expended in binge-ing and purging, many bulimarexic women manage to maintain high academic averages in college. By their own admission, they are overachievers. They tend to compensate for their perceived shortcomings by driving themselves, and when their talents are recognized they both thrive on and dislike the recognition ("I needed it to justify my awfulness and hated it because I felt undeserving"). However, the drive for academic success is often related to pleasing others and to the expectation of "marrying well" rather than to the personal joy of intellectual achievement. The expectation is that such achievement will lead to the fulfillments that marriage and childbearing can bring. For example, a doctor is more likely to meet and be attracted to a woman who is well educated; a woman is most likely to meet "her man" in a college or university. So achievement is seen mainly in terms of what rewards it can elicit from others, particularly men.

Most of these women describe themselves as never having had an intimate relationship with a man. Given their behavior, intimacy is difficult, if not impossible. Many continue to believe that social failure is due to their appearance and try to avoid dating altogether. Others become supremely critical of the men they encounter or adopt a clinging, possessive style with men who typically reject or otherwise abuse them. Even so, relationships with men are considered primary, and friendships with women, when they do exist, are often terminated when a man enters the picture. At best, relationships with women are likely to be superficial, since the bulimarexic is in constant competition with other women. She runs the risk of losing out on both counts.

This basically dishonest life style often leads to more

deviant behaviors. Not surprisingly, bulimarexics become adept at lying. Stealing is also frequent. They steal food from roommates ("I don't care if she's my best friend!"), family, and from stores and supermarkets. Some also steal money in order to restore depleted food supplies. Several women told us of having been arrested for shoplifting food. Confrontations with roommates or relatives over missing food supplies can lead to rifts and the kind of isolation that is the last thing the bulimarexic needs. One woman's story provides an example: "Sneaking food was always a great treat. I got to eat the food (first bonus) and nobody knew about it (second bonus). As an annual ritual my aunt baked Christmas pies several weeks before the holiday, and then froze them so we couldn't eat them beforehand. I snuck down to the freezer and ate them frozen! Unfortunately, I was caught and haven't been invited back."

Added to the bulimarexic's feelings of anxiety and shame is the sheer necessity of paying for the huge amounts of food consumed. Few women can afford the financial out-lay. For those who are married or living with families, this means outright stealing of money or ingenious camouflage of food bills (in addition to hiding evidence of binge-ing). It would not be an exaggeration to say that the cost of food for the bulimarexic could equal a large family's average food bill. Nicole, whose story began this chapter, would visit different stores each day so that replacement of food eaten in a binge would not be noticed. Another woman spent as much time devising ways of hiding food bills from her husband as she did binge-ing and purging. Major charge cards proved useful, because she could then make purchases at specialty stores in addition to grocery stores and supermarkets; the bills from each grocery store seemed smaller. For Nicole and other women like her, guilt becomes a constant companion (Nicole was literally "vomiting all the food my boyfriend and family worked so hard to buy"). And, sadly, energy that could be directed toward positive endeavors is dissipated in attempting to hide the bulimarexic behavior.

Some natural questions: What do these women get out of binge-ing and purging? What are the consequences? Are there rewards, payoffs? Ironically, it seems that there *are* for the bulimarexic, at least for the short term. Some describe binge-ing as a marvelous, albeit transient, release. This frenzied high inevitably leads to a more relaxed state; once they begin to binge, they report feeling calm. Since many bulimarexics report troubled sleep patterns and insomnia, they frequently use binge-ing as a kind of sleeping pill. Others describe the ecstasy of relinquishing control and surrendering to food. Some admit that their bizarre behavior makes them feel unique, gives them a feeling of specialness.

Purging then becomes a purification rite, a means of overcoming self-loathing by gaining self-control. Having reestablished their disciplined ways, the bulimarexics feel "good" and perceive themselves as the perfect human beings they strive to be. In describing the purge or the process of getting ready for the purge, some say they feel "completely fresh, clean again." A phrase often heard is "a new beginning." However, their feelings of self-worth are only temporary, and the fear persists that the binge compulsion will overwhelm them once again. It nearly always does. Since these women are convinced that they are unlovable and inadequate, they are extremely sensitive to even minor slights and frustrations, which will soon be used as an excuse to initiate another binge.

Rejection, confrontation, disappointments, and anxiety

are often major precursors of a binge. The decision to binge, more often than not, is related to the inability of bulimarexic women to assert themselves and deal with their problems in a direct way. Anger is a rare emotion for these women; they have been well socialized to be agreeable, compliant, and nonassertive. Their immediate response to disappointment and pain is to feel hopeless and helpless rather than angry. Most lack awareness of their inability to express anger and rationalize their need for control in a number of ways: i.e., "If I get angry, I will go completely crazy"; "If I allow myself to get angry and speak up, it will hurt other people"; "If I acknowledge my own human rights to be honest and angry, I will turn people off and be rejected." This sense of shame and guilt over their disordered eating pattern also effectively helps them to suppress anger. Thus, the action and problem solving that can follow the experience of anger and assertion—the very things that can result in productive change—are denied to most bulimarexics. They are stuck with the tried and true "feminine" way of dealing with pain and discomfort.

Bulimarexics report gorging and purging for some of the following reasons:

• As a way of avoiding failure. A woman may be anxious about writing a college term paper or making a difficult phone call. She may binge instead of taking action or may postpone taking responsibility by first binge-ing and then tackling the assignment that causes her anxiety. The student who flunks her exam may remark that she failed because she binged the night before rather than admitting that she failed because she did not prepare for the exam.
• As a way of handling the stress involved in new activities, particularly social encounters. The bulimarexic's

pattern of obsessional thinking allows her to separate from the person or people she is with at the moment. One woman expressed it this way: "I attended a party which included some well known people. As usual, I felt tongue-tied, dumb, and inconsequential. As usual, I smiled sweetly and engaged in chitchat. All the time I was secretly planning a midnight binge when I returned home." Another says: "I began binge-ing in order to alleviate the anxieties I had about undertaking new things, and to provide myself with an excuse to take a rest from everything once in a while."

• As a way of postponing sexual relations, as graphically expressed by the statement, "I'm too stuffed to want sex," or as a way of loving oneself when a sexual encounter is disappointing. The following statement is illustrative: "I say to myself, 'I love you (meaning me), even if *he* doesn't, so go ahead and *eat* if it makes you feel loved.' "

• As a way of eliciting attention and getting back at those people who the bulimarexic feels *made* her binge in the first place. This is, of course, the ultimate way of avoiding responsibility for the behavior.

The resolution to stop binge-ing forever is an important part of the cycle since it guarantees failure. Bulimarexics typically believe that total abstinence from forbidden foods is the only acceptable way of gaining control. Some are able to give up binge-ing for a considerable time—up to three or four months if their lives are running smoothly—but a rejection or even a minor disappointment can trigger a binge. Instead of congratulating themselves for what they have accomplished and acknowledging that they have made *one* mistake, they use the binge as an excuse for continuing as before. Having succumbed to one cookie or one piece of chocolate cream pie, they consider themselves out of control. The old "dieter's guilt," as one woman put it, takes over: "Since I've already blown it, why stop?"

Feeling themselves powerless in the moment, victims of near mystical forces that propel them toward uncontrolled eating, many women use a variety of techniques to aid themselves in their attempts to stave off binge-ing. They make endless lists of chores to keep themselves busy every minute of the day, keep journals, and write down complicated rules to which they must adhere. Some write inspirational notes to themselves, outlining resolutions and responsibilities. Others move from one strenuous diet to another. Still others literally move to a new apartment or job when the behavior becomes extreme. Thus, they delude themselves that they are "fighting" the behavior. Their days, which typically begin with good intentions and lists of things to do, usually deteriorate from control to chaos.

In time, the binge-ing and purging become habitual, and precipitating factors become irrelevant because binge-ing then occurs at any time and under any circumstance—when these women are happy, sad, excited, under stress, or depressed. The pattern has become an entrenched and crippling coping mechanism that is a major part of the bulimarexic's lifestyle.

The dilemma that results is well expressed by this woman: "It's easy to sit over an open half-gallon of ice cream and find solace in that—but it certainly is nowhere living."

CHAPTER 3

Socialization and the Family

Month after month we sit in a room with a group of very special women. They have vitality, talent, wit, and energy. The fact that they are also generally slim and attractive is quite secondary. What is primary—and tragic—is their inability to acknowledge their particular assets and their uniqueness. They are like championship thoroughbreds that wear blinders and run on circular tracks. Unlike thoroughbreds, however, they do not try to outrun their track-mates. Bulimarexics not only run on circular tracks with blinders, they also are too preoccupied with themselves to think about winning the race. In fact, they usually expect to lose! And, as we have seen, these women of high potential feel that the only way they can win is by being thin, thin enough to attain an ideal that might, just possibly, be unattainable. What has made them this way? What pressures make the women we treat feel that they should be paper dolls, all cut to one pattern?

Researchers and feminists have had much to say about these matters and have come up with a number of interesting conclusions, many of them centering around the socialization of women. While it is not possible for us to cover all these theories in this book, we do want to touch upon those that seem relevant to the women we are treating.

Until recently, it was thought that a woman could be fulfilled only as wife and mother. Whatever energies were left over could be devoted to volunteer activities or personal hobbies (generally undertaken without pay and in "spare time"). Women who sought to achieve in other areas were considered to be making adjustments that were substitutes for the feminine role. There were exceptions, of course. For reasons that have nothing to do with personal fulfillment, many women have had to work in order to augment family income. Others have gone against the grain of what was considered acceptable to pursue their own goals. But the tendency has been to view these women with a degree of alarm. The main goal for a woman was to appeal to and catch a man. After that, protected economically (and perhaps emotionally), the roles of wife and mother would involve her totally. The traditional boast of her husband was, "My wife doesn't work," and she subscribed to this notion as well.

As Susie Orbach has pointed out in *Fat Is a Feminist Issue,* "To get a man, a woman has to learn to regard herself as an item, a commodity, a sex object. Much of her experience and identity depends on how she and others see her." She attempts to conform to what "others will find pleasing and attractive" and also to what she *perceives* them to consider pleasing and attractive. The ideal woman, as presented in newspaper advertisements, in magazines, and on television—whether in commercials or in the programs themselves—becomes the ideal to which she should ascribe. Orbach goes on to point out how women are made to believe that "the body is not satisfactory as it is." The woman must deodorize and perfume it, bind it up or let it hang free, and scramble to renew the clothes that quickly become out-of-date according to the vagaries of fashion.

The feminine ideal itself has not remained constant throughout the ages. At times slimness has been prized, and at other times a certain degree of plumpness has received admiration. During some eras, the Victorian period, for instance, a modified version of *both* body types was desired simultaneously. Women of this time are pictured with ample hips and bosoms but with painfully constricted tiny waists. But no matter what the historical period, the common denominator for women has likely been the urge to conform.

In our own time, the exhortation has been for women to be thin. Certainly the fashion models in advertisements of forty years ago seem well cushioned in comparison with those to whom we are accustomed today. A careful perusal of the ads over the years will show us that models are becoming more and more emaciated, until an ideal that approaches anorexia exists.

Some researchers feel that extreme slimness is valued in industrial societies where food is plenteous. Others maintain that body ideal is related to the degree of freedom women enjoy in a particular era. For instance, Kim Chernin, in her book *The Obsession: Reflections on the Tyranny of Slenderness,* postulates that during periods of history when women are tied into their mothering and nurturing roles and are without personal power, they are "allowed" to appear more female, with emphasis on distinctive female characteristics (full breasts and hips). Conversely, in times when women are more liberated, the ideal of slimness, even boyishness, is in vogue. This could be seen in the twenties, when women joined the burst of freedom after World War I; and within the last decade, as women have made their way into the workplace in increasing numbers.

Along with the current pursuit of slimness, there has been a similar obsession with youth. Once mothers and daughters were distinguished from each other very clearly by their clothing. A mother's clothing reflected her maturity, or at least the maturity of her years. But fashions for both groups have become virtually indistinguishable, and it is not at all unusual for mothers and daughters to exchange clothes with each other. As Bess Myerson, once Miss America and now involved with public service, commented when this phenomenon took hold: "We used to dress like Jackie Kennedy, now we're dressing like Caroline."

The cults of slimness and of youthfulness were perhaps best personified by a young British model who first appeared on the American scene in 1966. Nicknamed Twiggy, and she did indeed resemble a twig, Lesley Hornby Armstrong was seventeen-years-old and at 5'7" weighed 97 pounds. Her hair was cropped, and her eyes, heavily made-up, gave her the appearance of waifishness. Soon her body, with its 31-22-32 measurements, caused a furor when it was featured in fashion magazine advertisements, and countless numbers of American women began to pattern their clothes styles, make-up, hair styles—and finally their bodies—after hers.

Today, Hilde Bruch, in *Eating Disorders: Obesity, Anorexia Nervosa and the Person Within,* and a number of other experts in the field of eating disorders point an accusing finger at Twiggy and feel that there is a correlation between her arrival in the United States and the appalling increase of diagnosed cases of anorexia nervosa. (The binge / purge syndrome as an eating disorder was still "in the closet" at that time.) Researcher Ann Beuf of the University of Pennsylvania also reminds us that the first outbreak of these disorders occurred directly after World War I, when the flapper type of woman was in style. One wonders if a person like Twiggy, singlehandedly as it were, could have established the trend in body type that has become so relentlessly pursued in recent years. Undoubtedly, the situation is more complex than that. However, Twiggy made her American debut at a time when the youth of America were a large and potent group of consumers. The baby boom infants, born after World War II, were adolescents, with their own money and their own power. Their numbers were legion, and their heroes were the mop-haired Beatles, the four young men from England who captured the American music scene and who looked like exuberant little boys.

So it might be said that young was in and slim was in; and big business hastened to cash in on both trends. The fashion industry formed and re-formed the ideal image (with variations on the same theme). During the unisex decade of the sixties, girls tended to look like boys and boys looked like girls—or, more accurately, both looked like little boys. Then, for both sexes, the long, thick bangs of the Beatles gave way to flowing locks. From the rear, it was often impossible to determine a young person's identity. And if the trend to wear trousers for all occasions seemed to imply freedom for women, there were certain aspects of fashion that continued to hamper them. In her book, *The Language of Clothes,* Alison Lurie notes the footgear for women wearing pants: stiletto heels, clogs, platform shoes. Throughout the book, Lurie assesses the history of female fashion as a "series of more or less successful campaigns to force, flatter or bribe women back into uncomfortable and awkward styles, not only for the purpose of vicarious ostentation and security of sexual ownership, but also and increasingly in order to handicap them in professional competition with men."

Another phenomenon appeared after the advent of Twiggy. The diet industry burgeoned into big business, catering to the national pursuit of slimness. Today, as we all know, it is impossible to turn on the television or to riffle through a magazine without having the "slim" message hammered at us. In spring diet articles appear like flowers, urging us to anticipate the bathing suit season. Even our social conversations invariably turn to diet groups, diet books, or the pros and cons of new diets that are currently being promoted. All of this has fed into—and continues to feed into—the consciousnesses of young women who believe that if they can conform to the ideal, be perfect in body, life's major problems will magically be solved.

Now let us examine some of the other aspects that enter into the socialization of women. It might be useful to run through a brief history of the mothers, and sometimes the grandmothers, of the young women we are treating for eating disorders today. For these young women, are the daughters of the first generation of women to have attended Weight Watchers. We will take a look at fathers as well.

During World War II, for reasons of patriotism and for money, millions of women (Rosie the Riveter) joined the labor force or various branches of the armed forces. When the war was over, it was assumed that most of them would relinquish their jobs in favor of returning veterans. The veterans themselves, with savings in hand and eligible for

Veterans Administration and Federal Housing Administration benefits, were eager to own their own homes. Newly married to young women, some of who were graduating from college in the forties and early fifties, they began the exodus to the suburbs. The nuclear family as we know it today became the American dream, with the husband / father who commuted to work in the city, the stay-at-home mother who tended the household and children, and the children who would receive all the benefits of fresh air and space and the privilege of growing up in a nonindustrial community.

Family life revolved around one father, one mother, and their children, with each family unit ensconced in a house that might be identical with or similar to other houses on the suburban scene. As generally happens after wartime, there was a trend toward larger families. With little or no household help and lacking the support of female relatives who might once have lent a hand with child rearing, young mothers—even those whose hopes for personal achievement might have been raised through college education—found it necessary to set aside individual concerns. Wives became chauffeurs for children and also for husbands who typically returned from the city at night or, in extreme cases, only on weekends. Feeling alone and isolated, yet indebted to their husbands for the economic security that made the dream of the suburbs reality, these women submerged themselves in the roles of wife and mother.

At first many were ecstatic, as Betty Friedan recalls in her book, *It Changed My Life: Writings on the Women's Movement:* "I felt that I would never again, ever, be so happy as I was living in Queens. The floors were parquet, and the ceilings were molded white plaster, no pipes, and the plumbing worked. . . . And now our friends were the other

couples like us, with kids at the nursery school who
squealed at each other. . . . It was fun at first, shopping in
those new supermarkets. And we bought barbecue grills,
and made dips out of sour cream and dried onion soup to
serve with potato chips, while our husbands made the mar-
tinis as dry as in the city and cooked hamburgers on the
charcoal, and we sat in canvas chairs on our terrace and
thought how beautiful our children looked, playing in the
twilight, and how lucky we all were, and that it would last
forever."

The media and big business had an investment in keeping women in the kitchen, at home, and in the role of consumers, and wondrous new appliances were manufactured
for their benefit—washers, dryers, and refrigerators in
decorator colors. The American housewife as the center-
piece in her gleaming kitchen was glorified. As Betty Friedan reminds us: in *It Changed My Life* "It certainly didn't
occur to any of us then, even the most radical, that com-
panies which made a big profit selling us all those washing
machines, dryers, freezers, and second cars were oversell-
ing us on the bliss of domesticity in order to sell us more
things. Even the most radical of us, in our innocence,
wanted those pressure cookers." The woman involved with
children, taking care of a home and a man, was made to
feel essential: "At home, you were necessary, you were
important, you were the boss, in fact—the mother—and
the new mystique gave it the rationale of career."

The feminine mystique, glorifying woman as mother and
homemaker, served to keep her complacent, satisfied, and
"lucky to have what she had." The small world of the
kitchen, nursery, and bedroom reinforced woman's traditional role as the caretaker who needed to be taken care
of.

However, as the decade of the fifties moved on, the picture changed. Many women began to wonder whether their suburban dream houses were prisons. Feelings of boredom, confusion, and meaninglessness emerged. When these women presented their "symptoms" to doctors, they were often given pills—to pep them up or calm them down—and told to buy a new dress or to devise new ways of satisfying their husbands and of gaining rewards from the mother/wife role. Experts advised the women to "escape" from the home for an occasional outing, failing to realize the extent of the problem. Many vulnerable women found the outings and pills insufficient. Midafternoon drinking provided relief, a phenomenon that increased to the point where sociologist Jessie Bernard concluded in *The Future of Marriage* that "the housewife syndrome might well be viewed as public health problem number one."

In 1957 Betty Friedan sent an intensive questionnaire to her college classmates, fifteen years after their graduation from Smith. Alarmingly, her classmates, the majority of who were middle-class housewives and mothers, described their lives as "incomplete" and "empty" and themselves as "almost non-existent." At the age of forty, they were questioning the meaning of their lives and regretting their decisions to give up or forego careers for marriage.

By 1963 Friedan had expanded her findings into a book she called *The Feminine Mystique,* and "the problem that has no name burst like a boil through the image of the happy American Housewife." It is difficult for young women of today to fully comprehend the confusion, excitement, and pain this book generated, as women realized that the problem that had no name was their problem too. Marlene was one of these women. Having completed her undergraduate work at the University of North Carolina, she had abandoned her dream of graduate school when her then husband decided to relocate in order to continue work on his Ph. D. Without questioning how it would affect her life, Marlene agreed to the move and to the need to help him complete his graduate training. This meant working as a salesperson in a department store, the only job available to a woman with a B.A. in fine arts in the city to which they moved. Twin daughters were born to her in 1963, followed by a son in 1965. Shortly after the birth of her son, as she cared for three children under three, Marlene read *The Feminine Mystique,* two years after its publication. Through tears, she realized that "she was not alone." With relief, she discovered that the anger, helplessness, and hopelessness that she was experiencing were shared by thousands of other women.

The Feminine Mystique galvanized women as it hit them where they were weakest, in the depths of their unawareness and passivity. In exploding the myth that all a woman needed to be happy was wifehood and motherhood, Friedan awakened a new wave of feminism that has helped to change society in important ways. She urged women to develop their own potential, to return to college and careers, and to fulfill themselves in meaningful work. At the time, this was a large order. Educational and career opportunities, particularly in the professions, were still denied to women. Discrimination against women worked in subtle ways, both in occupational settings and in universities. Financial aid, more often than not, was forthcoming for "putting the husband" through his education, but married women found themselves unable to compete for federal scholarships and loan aid because of the difficulty of managing both schooling and the home front.

There were, of course, many other women who had never developed skills or whose skills had become rusty during the years of homemaking. For these women, the frustration intensified. Although aware of the problem, they felt there was no place to go.

In the late sixties, the number of American women who were being psychiatrically "serviced" began to increase measurably. Pauline Bart, a sociologist at the University of Illinois, studied a large group of middle-class women who were patients in psychiatric hospitals. Suffering from what came to be called the "Empty Nest Syndrome," these women had become depressed when their children left home and were eventually institutionalized. Younger women with agoraphobia (the fear of being alone in a large open space) formed another distinct group in need of psychiatric help. As increased educational and occupational opportunities opened up, women with the aspiration but not the skills to cope with the responsibilities involved began to suffer from performance anxiety (a neurosis that had been thought to lie primarily in the realm of male psychiatric dysfunction).

Unfortunately, therapy often served to increase the women's sense of powerlessness and became an effective tool in further controlling them. There were few women therapists, and of those that there were, only a handful embraced a feminist orientation. Female patients, accustomed to male authority, preferred men therapists. Phyllis Chesler emphasizes this point in *Women and Madness:* "In 1960, the membership of the American Psychiatric Association totaled 11,083 of whom 10,000 were men and 983 were women. In 1970, their membership increased to 17,298 of whom 14,267 were men and 1,691 were women. Thus, 90 percent of all psychiatrists during the 1960's were men." In addition, many therapists, both psychologists and psychiatrists, were still rooted in psychoanalytic theory and accepted, lived out, and practiced stereotypical attitudes toward women in their own lives. Instead of directly addressing their patients' present and critical problems, therapists often redirected women's energy to the past and to intellectualizing rather than doing, acting, changing and growing in the present. Therapy was deemed successful when the "woman came to her senses" and got married or became pregnant. More often than not, therapy reinforced acceptance of the traditional female role.

This message, then, was transmitted to the daughters of these women. By and large, middle-class parents of the fifties were upwardly mobile, eager to provide their children with the material and intellectual advantages they may have felt they were denied. Often this meant a college education. However, expectations for male and female children were different. For young men, a college education was the ticket to career success and financial security. For women, the expected reward was marriage to a potentially successful, well-educated man, and it was important for women to "keep up with" their husbands. While young women might be praised for academic achievement during college, as the undergraduate years drew to a close, pressures increased to propel them toward popularity with the opposite sex and, eventually, an appropriate marriage. Well-intentioned parents wanted their daughters to be well taken care of, and the daughters themselves were eager for family approval.

In sum, as sociologist Lenore Weitzman points out in a chapter in *Women: A Feminist Perspective:* "The well-socialized American girl learns three clear lessons: one concerning her personality, a second concerning her capability, and a third concerning her future role. With regard to her personality, she 'knows' that to be truly feminine she will be sweet, expressive, not too intelligent, nurturing, cooperative, pretty, and fairly passive. With regard to her capability, she 'knows' she will always be less capable and less important than most men. With regard to her future, she 'knows' she will be a wife and mother. If she is a successful women, she will acquire this status soon. . . ."

During the sixties, the culture as a whole was experiencing a number of changes that caused upheavals in traditional attitudes and behavior. The civil rights movement attracted thousands of middle-class students and provided them with shocking revelations about life beyond their secure suburban communities. Other teenagers and students began to repudiate the materialism and "false" values of their parents and joined protests for an end to American involvement in Vietnam and for greater student control of education and free speech on campuses. Another contingency of young people broke away from their families to drop out as hippies, runaways, and flower children.

In addition to these revolutionary changes, the advent of oral contraceptives led to a "sexual revolution." With the fear of pregnancy virtually eliminated by the pill, women were encouraged toward a sexual openness that was once thought primarily the province of men. Young women might have intercourse with the men who they expected to marry, but premarital sex with a number of partners had not been the general rule. Now there was pressure to be freer, not to be "uptight and guilty," and for many women the so-called sexual revolution led to a new kind of anxiety. Multiple sexual contacts might give a temporary illusion of desirability, but women now experienced sex in ways that removed it from the realm of intimacy, security, and a feeling of connectedness. Beneath the freedom lay the conditioning to dependency that had characterized women, and the desire for a permanent connection remained. The lack of boundaries in relationships with the opposite sex often created new fears because suddenly nothing was predictable, and the comfort of familiar rules (and roles) appeared no longer to be there. This existential desperation drove many women to compete with each other more than ever for the attention of men, thus creating a self-consciousness about physical attractiveness and youth that was particularly intense. Here, again, advertisers and manufacturers found easy prey among these women preoccupied with being slim and young.

The decade of the seventies brought continued change for women. The burgeoning feminist movement resulted in women's consciousness raising groups and in a desire among women for increasing control over their bodies and their lives in general. New career opportunities opened up, and women were encouraged to express themselves with more assertion. But the pressures to succeed, along with heightened insecurity from unstable relationships, competition at work, and the increased incidence of divorce, took their toll. A number of studies conducted in the seventies indicated that under the cloak of feminism, the entrenched feminine modes of response remained. In many ways, women were talking like feminists, but continuing to act out the conventionally feminine fantasies and roles.

Barbara Ehrenreich and Deirdre English (in their book *For Her Own Good: 150 Years of the Experts' Advice to Women*) show that the slogan "You've come a long way, baby" was debatable. In pointing out that the seventies produced an ambiguous and frustrating form of liberation, they say:

"After the old dependency came the new insecurity of shifting relationships, a competitive work world, unstable marriages—an insecurity from which no woman could count herself 'safe' and settled. There was a sense of being adrift, but now there was no one to turn to. . . ." Socialization had conditioned many women to be dependent, passive, and noncompetitive, and they were unprepared for new roles.

It is not coincidental that the two uniquely feminine eating disorders—anorexia and bulimarexia—became widespread in the seventies and continue to engage our attention today.

Now let's take a closer look at the families of these women, with particular attention to the typical family constellation that can lead to the development of bulimarexic behavior.

"Mom is the villain." Overwhelmingly, this has been the conclusion whenever eating disorders in children are examined. Researchers and clinicians, and even feminist writers, are likely to hold mothers responsible; all deplore the controlling mother who is seen as "perfectionistic, domineering, and overinvolved" with her children.

This entrenched view is myopic, destructive, and unjust. In the area of eating disorders, mothers' overinvolvement in the lives of their daughters is rarely viewed as stemming from the same frustrations and feelings of helplessness and powerlessness that their daughters experience. Many experts evidence a total lack of compassion for these mothers, an almost self-righteous, across-the-board condemnation that fails to take into account the complexities involved in these mother-daughter relationships.

Typically, the mothers of our bulimarexics were women

who abandoned careers (or never embarked on them) in order to raise children. Initially, they glorified in their motherhood. The commitment to their families and homes was their means of personal fulfillment, and they subscribed to the view that children could not grow to full potential without a mother's constant attention and care. Like the college classmates Betty Friedan wrote about in *The Feminine Mystique,* these mothers made painful transitions into middle age. The vicarious gratification attained by way of a husband's achievement or the accomplishments of children no longer sustained them. Many grew increasingly disillusioned, depressed, and neurotic. Outwardly dominant, but inwardly weak and unhappy, these mothers felt ineffectual in most areas of their lives. Since they were married to men who were generally preoccupied with their careers, or "out to lunch," as one of our women put it, these mothers exercised "authority by default" over their children. At times they were suffocating and overbearing, as if to compensate for their powerlessness elsewhere.

Putting the blame on mothers may afford a certain satisfaction, in that mothers are punished for past trangressions, but it is especially destructive for bulimarexics. The young women then are focusing their energy on the past as they seek the underlying reasons for their compulsive eating habits. They are concentrating on the *whys* rather than on *what they are gaining* from such behavior patterns. Once women come to realize that they have embraced the same legacy of helplessness and hopelessness that their mothers have lived out, they can free themselves to choose a different way of living. They can reject what they perceive as frivolous, demeaning, and irrational, and can develop skills that are fulfilling and growth enhancing. The problem for many daughters is that in their attempts to move away from their mothers' legacy, they do not move toward other alternatives (except food). Daughters who cling to the belief that they are "tragic victims" who can only control their lives through food deny themselves the joys and pains of growth and the opportunity to develop competence, self-reliance, and independence. In blaming their mothers, they absolve themselves from personal responsibility and remain locked in the past, paralyzed in the present, and fearful of the future. They do not see their mothers as "victims" too and fail to understand or appreciate the pain and conflict that molded them.

Assuming the role of victim can have other disastrous consequences. Rather than rejecting the passive-aggressive behavior of their mothers, many of the bulimarexics we have treated struggle for a social acceptance that would allow them to reenact their mothers'· roles. Again, since they cannot imagine that there are alternatives, their only option appears to be to follow in their mothers' footsteps. The resulting and mutually demoralizing dependency results in further powerlessness for both mother and daughter. In overt and covert ways, the mother transmits her frustration at being a woman; the daughter, in turn, feels hopeless about her own future.

In our initial work with bulimarexic women, we too were caught up in stereotypical assumptions about mother-daughter strife, especially since many of our women were involved with struggles for independence. However, we soon learned that some of the women took issue with the condemnation of "mother as villain" and were upset by Marlene's first article about bulimarexia in *Signs,* which reiterated this theme. On the contrary, these women argued, they loved their mothers. In order to gain more

insight into these responses, we began to administer
detailed family history questionnaires to our group members and were surprised at what we learned. Taking into
consideration the bulimarexic's characteristic inability to
express open anger and the fact that she may not be able
to express her feelings honestly, there were nonetheless a
number of women who said they loved their mothers
unconditionally. Of the first 120 Cornell coeds polled, 55
percent characterized their relationships with their mothers as good. The following examples are typical:

"She has always had my interests at heart and tried to
teach me independence. She's strong and smart."

"Our relationship has been very close; she has been loving to all her children. I feel very much like her, and we
understand each other very well."

Others spoke of relationships, once stormy, that were
improving with time.

In addition to the 55 percent who described their relationships with their mothers as good, 40 percent said they
felt ambivalent. They both loved and hated their mothers.
On the one hand, they could respect their mothers for their
ability to juggle multiple roles and could admire their
physical beauty or social competence. On the other hand,
they had scorn for their mothers' weaknesses, rages,
and / or breakdowns. They swung from love to hate and
felt guilt during "hate cycles." Some even felt that they had
to protect their mothers from depression. The comment
of one woman sums it up: "If I start to live, she'll start to
die! Guilt! I was a great Mama's girl, very close. She is an
all-too-loving woman—she overparents me and is manipulative. I hate and love her. We fight a lot. She demands
to know my feelings and then tells me my feelings are
wrong. She's depressed a lot."

These women also resent the way their mothers submit to the domination of husbands: "After I became a teenager, I had little respect for my mother because I thought she would never stand up to my father." Another woman expressed herself in a similar way. The words she uses clearly illustrate her ambivalence: "We get along well, and we get along much better now than in the past. I do feel my mother lets my father dominate her too much. She works for him for no salary, and waits on him hand and foot. I love her, but feel sorry for her when she lets my father push her around."

In our experience, many bulimarexic women are likely to have approach-avoidance conflicts with their mothers. While they may despise their mothers at times and resent the suffocation of their overinvolvement, they nonetheless often seek their mothers' support. They love and admire them for certain qualities; they compete with them, feel sorry for them, and confide in them. In fact, the bulimarexic woman's relationship with her mother is often her only source of support in a closed and alienated nuclear family where the father is distant, either physically or emotionally or both.

For the most part, bulimarexic women do not express overt hostility toward their fathers. However, some of the same women who told us that they loved their mothers said that their fathers were the problem! It is interesting that few investigators have addressed the father's role in childhood disorders, particularly with regard to eating disorders. This obviously has to do with the status accorded the father's role as breadwinners who are preoccupied with their careers and who carry on the important and necessary work of men in the world outside the family. As Phyllis Chesler points out in *Women and Madness:* "Fathers invade children too (their privacy and selves, etc.), but not as frequently. They don't have to. They already own the entire territory and need only make occasional forays to check on their holdings."

The impact of these remote fathers can have far-reaching consequences for the family as a whole. Mothers generally take up the reins with bitterness when fathers relinquish their responsibilities. Although these mothers may appear dominant—at least in the home and over their children—they remain submissive to their husbands in all other realms. For it is the fathers who hold the economic bargaining power. And, as already indicated, the mothers exercise authority by default.

Paternal rejection and secret yearnings for intimacy with their fathers were evident in the history of many of the bulimarexics we treated. According to these daughters, lack of intimacy with their fathers was as much responsible for their feelings of inadequacy and lack of self-esteem as were the strife-ridden relationships with their mothers. A surprising 47 percent of our 120 coeds characterized their relationships with Dad as bad! Anger at him, when they were able to release it, was more vehemently expressed than that aimed at mothers. The following quotes illustrate the pain many women feel because of the unavailability of fathers:

"Daddy was always at work. Occasionally he noticed me. Usually he put me down. I hate him."

"Messed up! My father always traveled and was away more than he was home. He left us for two years to live in Europe."

"He is very reserved and never emotional. I can only communicate with him on a superficial basis. I have harbored deep resentment for my father and the pain he has caused my family."

Several women described their fathers as tyrannical and had always been frightened of their anger. One called her father "irresponsible, domineering and crazy. I stay away from him." Another said her father "rules the household with an iron hand. He's an autocrat, a little Hitler, we never talk." Others were fearful of the variability of their fathers' moods.

Occasionally, the daughters have some insight into how the behavior of father and mother feed into a family system that is damaging to all members. The daughter of a successful lawyer has this to say: "He will do anything for a client. As a father he leaves me empty. My father never hugs and kisses me. He hides his emotions and told me one had to hide one's emotions. My mother dropped out of college during her third year. A society belle, she married my father. There is no communication. We have a destructive relationship and I am ever dependent on them. They are my social life."

The following statement is even more perceptive: "My father is very insecure. He depends on his children to fulfill certain needs in his life and takes very personally the things that we do that may or may not fulfill needs in his life. He's very critical of me. My mother plays an interesting subordinate role but actually runs the family and is the dominant one. She allows my father to think that *he* does, however, because he needs to feel that."

In contrast to the closeness that had evolved over the years with mothers, many women felt that their relationships with their fathers were deteriorating. The high school or college years were pinpointed as the beginning of this

change for the worse: "We had a loving and trusting relationship until the last few years," one woman said, "I can
see through his idealistic crap now. He doesn't practice
what he preaches." While this comment might reflect the
young woman's general maturation, most women related
their conflicts with fathers to their first steps toward separation from the family. At this time, some fathers seemed
to want them to stay little girls or, at least, to accept the
traditional feminine role. Here are some indicative comments:

"For the most part, he favored me and loved me a lot
. . . but he turned away from me during adolescence. He
emphasized my looks, yet praised others for their mind
and talent."

"We got along together in high school, much better than
my mother and I, but since I've gone to college, my father
and I don't get along so well. He still treats me like a little
girl, but he'd like to see me get married."

"During high school he tried to make me into a female
domestic . . . after years of encouraging independence and
exploring interests!"

It might not be stretching it too much to say that these
fathers encouraged and supported their daughters while
they lived under the fathers' roofs, but once the young
women made efforts toward independence, fathers
encouraged them to become like their mothers.

Whatever criticism they had, many of the bulimarexic
women we questioned idolized their fathers. Fathers were
viewed as successful and powerful, and their attention and
approval, intermittent as it might be, was valued more than
the love they received from their mothers. When they felt
their fathers withdrawing, they often tried harder to please

them, usually without success. And so the ground was laid for the lifelong quest for male approval (often associated with physical perfection). This wistful statement from one of our women is indicative of the feelings of many: "My father is somewhat of a maverick—very successful and very much the outdoor sportsman and athlete. I tried so hard to emulate him and be his favorite."

Often the time when fathers withdrew from their daughters coincided with a move toward their growing sons. Another familial theme running through the histories of women with eating disorders is the intense competition they experience with siblings. Fifty-eight percent of the coeds sampled in our initial survey had older brothers and more often than not the brother was the favored child. Our women soon found that no matter how perfect or successful they were, the accomplishments of brothers were regarded more highly. They were learning "how to feel small," with the accompanying lesson that "good girls don't win ball games." What's more, the parental expectations for female and male children were quite different.

"Our parents had distinct aspirations for both me and my brother," one woman said. "He was encouraged to accomplish great feats in the world. I was just supposed to be happy, marry well, and love my children. There was the expectation he would pursue a career. It never occurred to them (or me) that I might someday have to support myself."

Some families discriminated in a more overt manner. In the following comment, when competition developed between a brother and sister, the girl was effectively muzzled, beginning at an early age:

"I have a brother who is fifteen months younger than I

am who at a very early age started to have psychological problems. A child psychiatrist told my parents that it was due to the fact that he was competing with me and I was always achieving. If something would break, I would fix it, for example. So, when I was about five or six, the psychiatrist told my parents that the competition was too much. I was deflating his male ego and they should try to separate us a little bit so that we weren't in competition so much. And the way my parents dealt with that was to tell me to try to stop doing better than him all the time. They asked me, don't fix it if it breaks, let him do it. They sort of asked me not to succeed and to succeed at the same time. From that time on, I've had the confusion of wanting to do well, but then being afraid that it wasn't okay to do well."

Thus we can see how maternal overprotection, paternal censure and deprivation, as well as rivalry with siblings (generally male) can propel a young woman toward the kind of stress that can result in eating disorders. We must, however, avoid the pitfall of relying on categories that are too neat, or we run the risk of creating new stereotypes. When we extended our initial treatment of bulimarexic college students to women of all ages and walks of life, we encountered many women who claimed that they loved and respected both parents. Their fathers, they said, were supportive and loving, and many of the mothers had achieved success in careers. Yet, although the family atmosphere had been more harmonious, these daughters typically had been overprotected. Most of them had not acquired the skills to cope with the world beyond the safe walls of the home. Raised to believe they were the "best," they learned to expect lavish praise and encouragement, but they had little experience with failure and rejection. And when they left home for college, their families were no longer there to envelop them with the protection they had grown to require.

Let us now turn to adolescence and the pressures that impinge on young women *outside* the family.

CHAPTER 4

Adolescence

SETTING THE STAGE FOR BULIMAREXIA

Seventeen magazine, in January 1982, featured an article entitled "Do You Stuff Yourself One Moment and Starve Yourself the Next?" The article introduced the magazine's readership, thousands of adolescent girls, to the binge / purge eating disorder. In a section of the article called "Where to Go for Help," our names were mentioned. Once again we received a dismaying number of letters. We no longer underestimated the epidemic nature of the syndrome and so were not particularly surprised at the amount of mail. However, to receive letters from girls who had not reached puberty—some of them only ten-years-old—gave us a new and shocking perspective!

One preteen told us with fear and even a bit of pride that her mother had not caught on yet to the fact that she made herself throw up four or five times a day "after eating everything in sight." Another girl, in her midteens, confessed that she had "bulimia, but not real bad." She had been vomiting once or twice a day for a year or so. A third complained, "No one will take me seriously. I know I am fat. Everyone says I'm just saying that to get attention, and they tell me I'm crazy." This girl added wistfully, "I guess they think I will outgrow it. I have tried to stop but can't."

For Marlene, the mother of teenage twin daughters, the letters were especially painful. She remembered all too clearly an incident that had taken place when Debbie and Becky were twelve. It was an incident that could have propelled the girls toward eating problems similar to the ones we are now writing about.

Marlene had always encouraged the twins to participate in sports, an experience she had missed when she was a young girl in the fifties. (At that time, boys typically engaged in strenuous physical activity, while girls dabbled at dance exercises and played volleyball.) At the age of twelve the twins had solid, trim bodies and were proficient in several sports. Gymnastics was the favorite, and they particularly liked their mother to watch them perform. Marlene literally wrote portions of her dissertation at the gymnastics center as the twins learned one routine after another.

At the end of the class, Marlene generally took the girls to the local Tastee Freeze for ice cream. One evening Debbie was very quiet, unlike her usual animated self, and said she did not want ice cream. No explanation. Marlene waited until they were home to ask what was wrong. Debbie dissolved in tears and said that she hated her body and wished she were dead: "I don't want breasts and I don't want hips. I hate my fat!" she sobbed.

Marlene was thunderstruck. As a feminist she had tried to help both girls develop a positive attitude toward their bodies and their emerging womanhood. Debbie was not fat, by any stretch of the imagination. Now, after treating numerous women suffering from bulimarexia, Marlene was seeing an anorexic-like response in her own healthy daughter.

After gentle prodding, Debbie revealed that her gymnastics coach had triggered her sudden loathing for her body. The coach had pointed to Debbie's stomach, slightly rounded as is normal for twelve-year-olds, and remarked, "You should lose a few pounds." That was all that was said.

Setting aside her role as therapist Marlene reacted emotionally as a mother. In detail she pointed out what she considered to be flaws and imperfections in her own body, and she told the twins that while she might not consider her body-type perfect, she would have to be satisfied with certain aspects of it for the rest of her life, no matter what self-restraint, no matter what amount of dieting. She asked the girls to love their bodies and accept the flaws and even invited them to consider her stretch marks, "created by the most beautiful experience I ever had, giving birth to twins."

It was a heady scene, with much crying and hugging, but afterward the girls appeared fortified and stronger. Four years later, Becky faced a similar experience, but handled it differently. She was trying to earn a much-coveted spot on the gymnastic team, and to her delight was chosen. Becky was then 5'3" and weighed 110 pounds. Her new coach immediately indicated that she would have to lose from 10 to 15 pounds. Without hesitation, Becky told the coach that losing that much weight would weaken her body and interfere with her performance. She quietly indicated her refusal and quit the team.

Such experiences, unless properly handled, indicate how an irrational fear of being fat can develop. Indeed, the preference for thinness can begin to take hold at a much earlier age, reflecting the preferences of our culture.

In 1978 researchers at the University of Cincinnati College of Medicine examined the attitudes and preferences of preschool-age children in an effort to find the age at which antifat concepts emerge. Overwhelmingly, most (91 percent) preferred a thin rag doll over a fat one. The handful of overweight children in the study also chose the thin doll, although they could not say why. As early as three- to five-years-old, then, there is a certain stigma attached to being overweight, and selective pressures on female children may have already been implanted. Other long-standing childhood studies support the findings that children develop a distinct aversion to chubby bodies and prefer athletic lean ones. In 1967 Dr. J. R. Staffieri of the University of Indiana presented six- to ten-year-old male boys with silhouettes of obese, normal, and thin bodies. Uniformly, the subjects reacted unfavorably to the fatter ones. Furthermore, they attributed disparaging characteristics to the "fatty," labeling it as dirty, lazy, lying, sloppy, mean, ugly, and stupid. In 1972 Staffieri showed the same silhouettes to female children. They too reacted unfavorably to the fatty, but added even more negative characteristics to their descriptions of it.

So it seems that both boys and girls disparage fat in childhood; however, beginning with adolescence, females overwhelmingly become more influenced than males. In 1971 Dr. E. Clifford at the Duke University Medical School found that 194 adolescent females aged eleven to nineteen were more dissatisfied with and critical of their bodies than 146 males of the same age range. A later study at the University of Iowa revealed that girls were beginning to undergo a distortion of body image, believing that they looked quite a bit heavier than they were. Eighty-six girls (ages ten to eighteen) from the Iowa City schools consistently overestimated the girth of their bodies. These studies indicated that young females wanted to be smaller but believed themselves incapable of attaining this deal. Many experts in eating disorders believe these early childhood attitudes persist and may contribute to self-loathing and poor self-esteem in those who gain weight at later ages and could create extreme self-consciousness in anyone who fears becoming overweight.

The cultural message to be slim is transmitted to the child through many sources—the family, the child's peer group, teachers, books, magazines, and television. Children try to behave in a way that is consistent with the beliefs and behaviors of people in the groups to which they belong. When all groups agree, certain values are introjected without question. In our culture, the message is clear: slimness is best.

At the same time, there is much to encourage excessive eating and weight gain. An abundance of fast food products exists, and we are bombarded with manipulative advertising from the food industry. Junk foods and fast foods are described as luscious and mouth-watering, with consumers challenged to binge: "Bet you can't eat just one!" Tempting snack foods help us to chew away our leisure hours. The presence of food is tied to recreational events and socializing, with cookouts, clambakes, and picnics part of the "American way of life." We are led to snack during movies or while watching television. Children and teenagers are especially susceptible to this kind of advertising.

If both boys and girls disapprove of fat in childhood and yet experience simultaneous conflicting messages to be slim and to eat excessively, what happens in adolescence to escalate this hatred of fat and self in girls? The answer seems to lie in the socialization rituals to which both sexes, but particularly women, are exposed. What are these socialization rituals and how are they conveyed? What are the subtle as well as overt pressures that encourage smallness of mind and body in adolescent girls?

Adolescence has always been an emotionally difficult passage, with youngsters typically feeling isolated, different, and out-of-step. Dr. Peter Blos, author of several books on adolescent passage, views this stage of life as a "struggle to regain a psychic equilibrium which has been jolted by the crisis of puberty." Blos believes the basic task of the adolescent is to arrive at a subjective feeling that "this is my way of life." A failure to achieve this sense can lead to adaptive failures and even severe psychopathology. Erik Erikson stresses these same major points in his developmental theory.

In our culture, the problem is that "identity" involves different goals and expectations for boys and girls as they move away from their primary identity of child and toward adolescence. Caryl Rivers, Rosalind Barnett, and Grace Baruch emphasize this point in their book *Beyond Sugar and Spice: How Women Grow, Learn and Thrive.* "Boys aim high—they look at the stars. Girls seem to peer up to the lowest branch in a nearby tree" (and, we might add, cling to it for dear life). For boys, signposts along the road to masculine identity have always been clear and well defined. "To be a man" implies strength of character, courage, and the willingness to take risks and become independent. Until recent years, "To be a woman" meant serving and caring for other people. Men were taught to be outwardly directed and "to make a go of it" before settling down and taking on new responsibilities and obligations. Men have been conditioned to move away from their original families and to find primary fulfillment through work. Women, on the other hand, have been directed away from their families of birth to form new families in which caring for husbands and children has been expected to provide the ultimate fulfillment. In *Beyond Sugar and Spice,* the authors sum up adolescent passage as the time when boys become men by doing and girls become women by finding a man.

Self-concept evolves through social interaction and is largely a product of socialization. There is now evidence that parents, especially fathers, regard their male and female infants in different ways based solely on the infant's gender. Although infant girls may weigh more at birth and actually be more hardy than comparable boy infants, they are still viewed as weaker and more fragile.

When children enter nursery school, teachers often react differently to boys and girls. One study of nursery school children reported that girls were encouraged to cling and ask many questions, while boys were taught to do and to be active. Other researchers report a sharp rise in "people orientedness" among girls at about the age of ten. Throughout adolescence, girls are more dependent than boys on the favorable opinions of others. Self-consciousness (as opposed to a sense of self) increases in girls and decreases in boys as they begin to mature.

Success experiences in adolescence are, of course, crucial in developing a sense of confidence and self-esteem. However, researchers have found that girls begin to value *interpersonal success* more than boys at this time. Girls depend so much for their identities on relationships with others, especially boys, that rejection can be devastating. Boys certainly experience rejection in relationships, but they are in the process of forming identities that can sustain them. The young male is admonished to "act like a man" when disappointed and to "pick himself up" and carry on. By the time boys reach adolescence, they have had much more experience dealing with criticism, defeat, and rejection. Witness any typical adolescent dance! The boys are lined up on one side of the dance floor, the girls on the other. The twelve-year-old boy ventures across the floor as his male friends watch carefully. When he reaches the chosen girl, he asks her to dance. She refuses. Amidst the hoots and jeers of his peers, the young boy must traverse the endless distance back to his friends. He may feel "little and small' but he does not "act it." His socialization has already taught him that men do not allow themselves to be brought down by such experiences.

Girls, on the other hand, are reinforced for dependent and approval-seeking behavior. With little experience in developing confidence and autonomy, they carry a greater fear of rejection than do boys. This fear, when combined with an obsessive preoccupation with boys, can become a prominent and primary psychological characteristic of adolescent girls, leading to irrational and crippling fantasies about their own fragility, helplessness, and powerlessness. Confidence in being able to cope with their environment is thus eroded by such paralyzing fears and expectations related to the horrors of "rejection."

In almost all aspects of a young woman's life, then, the answer to "what is my identity?" is fraught with negative associations. The period of adolescence for women has been described as a "dropping back" time, a turning away from individual achievement and competition toward what Jean Lipman Blumen, of the National Institute of Education, describes as "the Vicarious Achievement Ethic." Perhaps this settling for less was revealed in an important 1978 study conducted by John C. Condry and Sharon L. Dyer of Cornell. Sixty-one children in the fifth, seventh, and ninth grades were given what were described as intelligence tests. Boys were assigned girl partners and were seated across from them. Each boy and girl was then taken aside and each was told that he or she had done better than his or her partner: "You won—you were five points better!" The youngsters were then given a second chance at the test. The researchers had set up this situation to test what they predicated would be a "sudden onset" of fear of success among girls in *mixed sex* competition at the time of puberty—the time when beliefs about "sex appropriate" behaviors are apparently formed. The results were illuminating. Both male and female fifth grade students increased their scores on the test the second time around. However, between the fifth and seventh grade, a radically different pattern emerged. Seventh grade boys increased their scores, while 80 percent of the girls dropped their scores after being told that they had bested a male partner. To a lesser degree, the same was true for the ninth grade girls. When they were asked about their test responses, most seventh grade girls—those at the onset of puberty— revealed a reluctance to compete with boys, especially to beat them at games. One ray of hope lay with the second group of ninth grade girls, who did not drop their scores. They felt they should always try their best no matter what the circumstances!

One other important aspect of adolescence that must be mastered is the ability to form new and more mature relationships with one's own age group. Here again current research suggests that adolescent friendships among males reinforce movement toward activity and achievement while girls, fearful of being on their own, tend to cling to each other. While boys use friends as allies in efforts to break away from authority, girls often form intense conformist alliances, which researcher Janet Lever has referred to as "mini marriages." Much of their conversation centers around how to snare this boy or that one—in short, there is an excessive, often obsessional, amount of thinking about boys.

Identity is often described by contemporary social scientists as *the things one does,* and the need is emphasized for several identities—some vocational and some recreational. The amount of success experienced in each of these identities determines self-concept. When successes outnumber failures, there is a reasonable chance that a positive identity will be formed. If a young girl's identity is so closely tied to successes in interpersonal relationships (which are typically transient and short-lived at this age), it is not difficult to see how the adolescent girl can develop a negative or "nothing" identity. Brothers and boyfriends are, of course, extremely interested in girls, but their energies are directed into other pursuits as well. They are forming a positive attitude toward their growing bodies by developing them and feeling the strength and power of their maleness. This positive acceptance of one's body is also consistently cited as another crucial developmental task to be mastered in adolescence. While boys may find the changes in their bodies as disturbing and disorienting as girls do the changes in their own, they rarely view these changes as crippling or subtracting from their self-concept—quite the contrary, as Rivers and her colleagues point out, they are "badges of manhood."

A special rite of passage for women involves the onset of menstruation. There is ample evidence that adolescent girls, even today, have negative feelings about their bodies as they begin their menstrual cycle. A major study conducted in 1978 by Anne E. Clarke and Diane Ruble of Princeton found overwhelming evidence that both female and male adolescents entertain very negative beliefs about menstruation. Over 50 percent of the girls worried that someone would know they were having their periods. Further, both sexes equated menstruation with emotionality and with disruption of activities as well as performance in school. Judith Bardwick, a psychologist at the University of Michigan, begins an essay about women's psychological conflict and the reproductive system by stating: "To a very large extent women are their bodies." It would not be too extreme to add that women become "prisoners of their bodies" as well. The following is a beautiful but unfortunately rare attempt on the part of one family to reverse these crippling socialization rituals. In her book *Menstruation and Menopause,* Paula Weideger cites a letter she received from parents: "We have two daughters, twelve and seven. The twelve-year-old just had her first menstruation. We drank wine and toasted her. Her father gave her a bunch of wild flowers. She seemed pleased and open."

In our view, the general inability of adolescent girls to take pride in their bodies is one important reason why they have great difficulty establishing identities as women. Few realize that females are more durable physically than males. Consider that the female must be strong enough to nourish and carry the fetus through the prenatal period in order to insure the survival of the species. During the course of evolution, it is hypothesized that stronger females survived, while males, whose role in procreation does not require that kind of strength and endurance, were not selected for those qualities. The *myth of feminine fragility* must be banished and young women must learn to identify positively with their bodies. This includes accepting and embracing changes that take place in the body. The bloating and weight gain that often accompany menstruation need not be viewed as unbearable. The pregnant female body, often associated with "unattractive changes" and the belief that "I will never have a perfect body again," should engender feelings of joy, power, and uniqueness, not self-loathing.

Emerging sexuality can also create enormous conflict in young women and increase the fear and distrust they have about their bodies. While they may be physically capable of the sexual act, few are ready for it emotionally. Our current mores present special problems. No longer is there the proscription to "save one's virginity." The so-called sexual revolution of the sixties did away with this important psychological protection. (To be fair, it was a proscription accepted by young men as well, at least as far as the "girls they were going to marry" were concerned.) Today, the pressure to have early sexual experiences is intense and unrelenting. Understandably, many young women begin to think of themselves as victims. This feeling coincides with the time when they are beginning to receive special attention because of external attractiveness. All around, there are pressures that perpetuate the image of woman as ornamental, with her body the main commodity of worth. And behind this is the ultimate fantasy of attracting and capturing a man. Thus, "going along with him" and the "fear of losing him" can create overwhelming anxieties. The young girl is already learning to adapt to the desires and needs of others and, in effect, makes her own transformation into a sexual object.

Advertisements further convince us that this is how women are or want to be. According to sociologists Gloria I. Joseph and Jill Lewis, advertising creates and shapes our values and fears so that we come to believe that imposed values / fears / attitudes / goals are our own, as if we had chosen them. In 1982 Joseph and Lewis conducted a survey of leading women's magazines to determine how female sex roles are presented and portrayed and to explore recurrent themes. They found that beauty ads comprised 68 percent of all advertising in *Cosmopolitan* magazine, and most women were portrayed as sexy, subordinate, and seductive, as competitors with other women, and as dependent on men. These researchers concluded: "The purpose of such institutionalized sexism operates in advertising for the purpose of maintaining the image of women as dependent sex objects who are inferior and subordinate to men. Consumerism is therefore promoted by keeping women in a constant state of self-doubt and self-denigration. They are constantly admonished to aspire to impossible standards of beauty and sexuality by *spending*. The selling of the image of woman as a sex object is big business and results in women competing against one another to achieve this illusionary image."

In 1977 sociologist Erving Goffman of the University of Pennsylvania observed that advertisements tended to show men as physically elevated above women, therefore reinforcing the image of women as deferential and dependent. In order to pursue these findings further, in 1978 Dane Archer and his associates at the University of California at Santa Cruz examined a total of 1,750 published photographs from *Time, Newsweek, Ms.,* and a number of newspapers. They found a pronounced tendency in all publications to emphasize the faces of men and the bodies of women. Their conclusion was that this was a clear reflection of the tendency to slight the intellectual qualities of women.

Since childhood, female children have been exposed through schoolbooks to portrayals of women in ways that are stereotyped and limited. In 1972 Lenore Weitzman and her colleagues at Yale conducted a study of award-winning preschool picture books and concluded: "Little boys receive attention and praise for their achievements and cleverness. For girls, achievement is marriage and becoming a mother. Most of the women in picture books have status by virtue of their relationships to specific men—they are wives of the kings, judges, adventurers and explorers, but they, themselves, are not the rulers, judges, adventurers and explorers. Through picture books, girls are taught to have low aspirations because there are so few opportunities portrayed as available to them. . . . Women . . . can achieve only by being attractive, congenial and serving others."

Educator D. B. Graebner studied 500 stories presented in elementary school readers over a ten-year period and reported similar findings in an article published in 1972. Men and boys outnumbered females in the newer editions and role stereotypes were, if anything, *stronger* in spite of the new feminist awareness of the sixties and seventies. Boys continued to be portrayed as clever, brave, creative, and resourceful, while girls were docile, kind, dependent, and self-abrogating.

Television has become a major influence in the lives of children and also a major means of transmitting the values of society. Many social scientists are quick to point out that the recent wave of feminism has had an impact on television programming, and we can observe it, too. Women are now portrayed as doctors, lawyers, even truck drivers, and display strength of character and courage. However, many commercials continue to portray women as insipid, mindless creatures, which may subtract from the influence of the new models of womanhood. Certainly, the commercials for such merchandise as jeans carry a promise of all good things if the wearer is slim and a threat of failure if she is not.

Additionally, program material on television continues to reinforce a terror of being fat. Well-known actresses who over the years have appeared in movies and on television are significantly slimmer today. Some even appear too thin and unhealthy. Recently, we watched several segments of the Johnny Carson show. Almost without exception, when women were conversing with each other, the focus was on dieting and the need to lose weight or on weight-related matters. One newly arrived South American singer remarked that she had left the poverty of her country for the United States "in order to eat." Now, after considerable struggle to get here, she had discovered that "she cannot eat!"

Drs. Susan and Orland Wooley, experts on obesity at the University of Cincinnati Medical School, have commented about a television commercial that depicts a fat woman bludgeoning her meek husband with her purse because he did not buy a motorcycle. In another sequence, a macho man who did buy one rides by with a slim young woman clinging to his back. They use this example to illuminate how fat people are ridiculed and ostracized by the media. Occasionally, a more compassionate portrait of an overweight person does find its way to the T.V. screen. However, the compassion conveyed is often dissipated by the simplistic behavior of the characters, who are usually always stereotypes. Such was the case with "Dinky Hocker," an ABC afterschool television special about an obese adolescent girl, which was shown several years ago. Dinky had friends who genuinely cared about her, including boys. She also managed to have fun in social situations. Predictably, however, she dealt with her discomfort about her obesity by overachieving academically and filling her life with hobbies and animals.

Although the film captured Dinky's life in a sensitive and realistic way—i.e., you genuinely felt Dinky's pain and liked her—it was superficial and myopic. From the onset, there was no doubt that it was all Mom's fault. Dinky's mother was portrayed as vicious, obsessed with her life as a committee woman, preoccupied, domineering, overbearing, hysterical, and unfeeling. She referred to Dinky's excess weight as "baby fat" and pushed food on her when she was attempting to diet; she interfered with and effectively sabotaged Dinky's first relationship with a caring boyfriend; she persisted in calling the girl Dinky instead of using her real name, Susan; and she ignored Dinky's weak and pathetic requests for more time and attention. Dinky almost always turned to food after some rejection or confrontation with her mother.

Dinky's father was weak, kindly, passive, and ineffectual. He basked in the glow of his wife's community efforts and spent most of his time as a referee between mother and daughter. While it is clear that he was distant and remote from Dinky, as was her mother, the film gave little indication that there was anything lacking in the quality of this father-daughter relationship. His problems with Dinky were never explored or challenged. Rather, the film appeared to accept his passivity unconditionally.

After a major crisis in the family, Mom came to her senses and realized that Dinky's pain was all her fault and that she had better stay home with Dinky where she belonged. The film ended with mother and daughter embracing, as Dad stood by, smiling in his casual, benevolent way.

Along with such antiobesity propaganda, there are extraordinary cultural persuasions to diet. We have come to believe that all life's problems can be solved by dropping pounds. Promises of success, transformation, an end to existential pain, and living happily ever after prevail. Myriad women (and some men) make a fetish of being thin and follow one reducing diet after another without knowing or caring that they can do so only at the price of severe anxiety and persistent health problems. Until very recently, being underweight was not considered as dangerous nutritionally as being overweight. Dr. Hilde Bruch believes that chronic malnutrition resulting from an abnormal preoccupation with weight is common but not readily recognized as abnormal because it appears under the guise of desirable slimness. Medical experts are only now beginning to call attention to the health hazards of indiscriminate or fad dieting.

In an editorial for the *International Journal of Eating Disorders* (Spring 1982), entitled "The Beverly Hills Eating Disorder: The Mass Marketing of Anorexia Nervosa," the Wooleys provide a scathing indictment of this best-selling popular diet. Pointing to the serious medical problems that can occur if this diet is followed, they say: "That training in anorexic psychopathology is selling so well holds a message. It is a vote of no confidence in the whole effort by helping professions . . . and it reveals a degree of desperation heretofore unknown. The figures mean that women are so afraid of fat they are no longer willing to wait for a safe scientific method of weight control. . . . The prevailing belief is that no price is too high for thinness, including health."

Jane Brody, health columnist for the *New York Times*, has also spoken out about the dangers of the Beverly Hills Diet and other fad diets. Unfortunately, such condemnation does not appear to budge these books off the best seller lists, and they proliferate.

With the insidious linkage between attractiveness/ success and dieting, it should not be surprising that even young women without severe interpersonal problems become preoccupied with weight in adolescence and engage in competitive and contagious dieting regimes with other young women. For adolescence is the time that the pressure to become popular with boys and to appear feminine is greatest. The implicit cultural belief is that there *must be something wrong* with a girl who gains weight, even though it is not at all unusual for both boys and girls to have some weight gain during adolescence. If youngsters are active and do not develop severe anxiety over the weight gain—which fosters the urge to binge—most of them would lose weight in a gradual and safe manner in a relatively short period of time. The exhortation to lose weight comes at a time when food becomes an important aspect of social life (think of pizza parties and clambakes, for instance), creating additional tensions beyond the usual anxiety about heterosexual relationships. All of this can keep a adolescent from enjoying new social experiences in a relaxed and easygoing fashion.

When the concerned parents of an adolescent girl consult physicians or books about overweight and dieting, they may find a reiteration of many of the opinions and beliefs that drove their child to strenuous dieting in the first place. Lest the story of Marlene and her twin daughters seem like an isolated instance, consider the following article, which appeared in the *New York Times* in December 1981. Here a school system and consulting physicians (save one) join hands to reinforce the pursuit of slimness as the ideal.

FAT GIRLS LOSING OUT ON SCHOOL DRILL TEAM

Great Falls, Mont., Dec. 19 (AP)—A curriculum committee has voted to keep fat girls off a high school drill team, unless they can show they are losing a pound a week.

The ruling, which supported school policy, was made last week, despite an appeal from a parent of a Great Falls High School student who said some girls were drinking mineral oil and taking other drastic measures to lose weight.

One girl, in tears, told the school board committee, "If you don't have a weight problem, you just don't understand." But she admitted that she had not followed the 1,500-calorie diet recommended by Eileen Solberg, adviser to the drill team, the Bisonettes.

Three physicians sent the committee a letter supporting the rule, but a fourth, Dr. Daniel Molloy, said the weight restrictions could be dangerous. He said the pressure placed on the young girls by peers and teachers could result in health problems as they tried to lose weight.

As we can see, overweight is still viewed as "the problem," without regard for the frame of mind or underlying issues that led to the overweight—*if there were any to begin with!*

The bulimarexic women we have worked with describe a variety of different pressures that led to their first decision to diet. A majority were overprotected and unprepared for the new demands posed by socializing with the opposite sex. Their families were self-contained units and the girls, as adolescents, felt isolated and socially insecure.

Significantly, few were actually overweight at the time. One woman describes how she felt prior to her first diet: "I was a junior in high school, very desperate—longing for a boy-friend. I had a shallow social life—lived in a fantasy world—had faraway crushes that never materialized, but even so, always felt that I wouldn't be able to handle them if I did. Somehow I believed a loss of eight pounds would magi-cally transform me into the princess."

The wish for magical personality transformations are often associated with expectations of weight loss. Shyness, feelings of inadequacy, confusion about men, and even ignorance will disappear as each pound is shed. The ado-lescent girl hopes that a new personality will be handed to her without any effort on her part. Sleeping Beauty will be awakened by a kiss!

Many women also say that a rejection (generally by a boy) in adolescence was the traumatic event that precipi-tated their first diet. More often than not, however, the adolescent girl *fantasizes* that she has been rejected because she is too fat. Most actually never heard this from the boys who had rejected them. For example, the two women whose words follow are certain that their fat resulted in rejection even though they had no real proof that this was the causal factor:

"My first real boyfriend dropped me without any expla-nation. All I felt then was rage at myself for being so fat and ugly and I vowed never to be that way again."

And the other says, "I had a boyfriend who dropped me inexplicably and I tied it to being fat."

Pressures can also emanate from family members. Mothers who are themselves obsessed with dieting may express horror when their daughters gain a few pounds:

"My mother made me very conscious of my chubbiness after my last summer at overnight camp (age thirteen). I gained nine pounds and was made to feel ashamed and guilty."

Fathers, too, can set the wheels in motion. although their total time spent with daughters may be less than in the mother-daughter relationship, their influence is powerful. Many times their standards of attractiveness for daughters are high, and a chance comment such as "you've put on a little weight" can create a humiliating sense of inadequacy in girls. As one young woman, who desperately wanted to please her father, put it: "Ever since I can remember, I wanted to be thin. Thin was in and fat people just weren't as attractive. I thought my thin cousin was somehow better because she was so slender, and I can remember standing behind her in grade school wishing my legs (which were normal) were as thin as hers. I was absolutely traumatized at age fourteen when my father told me I had a fat ass. Somehow I think I just always wanted to be Daddy's daughter and couldn't bear the thought of losing loving nicknames such as 'little face" or 'little bit.' "

The overwhelming desire to please others coupled with extreme self-criticism is the essence of the problem. Debbie and Becky were especially vulnerable to this type of criticism because they were athletes. A similar vulnerability is evident in young dancers. Dr. L. M. Vincent, author of *Competing with the Sylph: Dancers and the Pursuit of the Ideal Body Form,* is a physician (also a dancer) who has observed many impressionable young dancers forced by the weight obsessive dance subculture into destructive eating patterns. In his book, he describes his anger, frustration, and surprise at seeing a young slim dancer he delights in—

"about the healthiest little girl I know"—reduced to tears and instilled with an intense desire to diet by the casual criticism of a dance coach:—"Watch your weight."

Once dieting is initiated, the process and the end result become as important as the factors that led to the diet in the first place. Dieting provides a sense of meaning and purpose—a distraction from pain, loneliness, and insecurity. Many girls derive feelings of power from this form of self-denial. Others derive secondary gains for their vigilance. Friends are admiring and in awe of the self-denial required to lose weight. "Gee, you've lost a few pounds!" can create temporary feelings of self-esteem. There are often negative consequences as well. In their dieting efforts many young women begin to harbor obsessive, selfish, and competitive feelings toward other women, gloating secretly when others are overweight. While they may want friendship, their preoccupation with body and their shyness keeps them from gaining friends (or from being a good friend themselves)

The way the adolescent girl deals with the disillusionment and unfulfilled expectations about weight can be crucial. The following account casts light on how the feelings of despair and emptiness following dieting attempts can facilitate bulimarexic behavior:

"I guess I started feeling down about myself and my weight in seventh grade. I was about five feet tall and weighed 120 pounds. Since no boy would want to 'go out' with Minnesota Fats (one of my nicknames), I became the matchmaker for everyone. I was the one a boy would call up if he liked one of my friends. I was also the one who would be called if someone needed a homework assignment. Furthermore, I was the one who helped plan the dances and then spent the night sitting on the garbage can in the girl's locker room. I played the part of the class clown, thinking that if I made people laugh they wouldn't care if I was fat. Finally, at the end of ninth grade, I decided to do something about my weight. I lost 10 pounds and grew two inches. . . ."

This young woman goes on to describe the anger and confusion she felt upon discovering that her weight loss brought her no greater social success. She returned to being "social chairman" and "good ole girl" and slowly gained back all her weight and then some. Soon after, she initiated the binge / purge cycle that was to cripple her life for thirteen years. Such unrealistic and unfulfilled expectations about weight are crucial in the subsequent development of both anorexia and bulimarexia.

Why do some young women choose bulimarexia and others anorexia? The major clues may lie within the family. Those who are not overly dependent upon their families and who have made some successful steps toward personal identity seem less likely to resort to anorexia. Even though the young woman described above was lonely and unhappy in many ways, the fact that she continued to move through her social world in a competent manner may be significant. Her role as "clown," although painful, meant that she had friends and, therefore, some self-esteem.

It may be that the younger the woman, the more socially isolated and family bound, the greater the chance she will develop anorexia as a means of controlling her environment and / or punishing her family. At this critically painful time in her life, the anorexic makes an overstatement to the world (primarily to her family) about her misery and feelings of inadequacy. Her starving body screams out for nurturing and attention. The bulimarexic, on the other hand, embarks on a harlequin existence, hiding her pain and loneliness and living in dread that her "disgusting" habit will be exposed. She is not retreating from the challenges and responsibilities of being a woman, as the anorexic is, but is trying too hard to conform to the feminine ideal.

If she manages to survive the agony of these adolescent years, there is another traumatic period that may very well propel her toward one or the other of these eating disorders. This is the period when she makes the important break from her family, home community, and school, and enters college or begins a career.

CHAPTER 5

The College Years
and Beyond

In 1946 Mirra Komarovsky, a sociologist, surveyed female students at Barnard College in order to assess the various academic and social pressures they were experiencing. Many of these young women admitted to being confused about conflicting expectations from family and other relatives. One student stated her dilemma as follows: "Uncle John telephones every Sunday morning. His first question is: 'Did you go out last night?' He would think me a grind if I were to stay home Saturday night to finish a term paper. My father expects me to get an A in every subject and is disappointed by a B. He says I have plenty of time for a social life. Mother says that 'A in Philosophy is very nice dear, but please don't become so deep that no man will be good enough for you.'" Komarovsky's studies were conducted over forty years ago. Optimistically, we would imagine that the impact of the women's liberation movement has eliminated more traditional standards of feminine behavior and encouraged independent achievement for women. However, if Komarovsky had visited a college campus today and polled its female students, she would have been surprised to find responses almost identical to those of her 1946 survey. The paradoxical messages from family and society as a whole have continued with distressing persistence. On the one hand, the young women are expected to excel academically, to be attractive, and to have an active social life; on the other, they are encouraged to remain "invisible," which translates to mean not too self-reliant, assertive, or serious.

The middle-class bulimarexic women who began to fill our therapy groups appeared even more protected, helpless, and desperate for male approval than their 1946 counterparts. In addition, they were overwhelmed by concerns about physical appearance and the pursuit of slimness. Joanne, one of our initial Cornell group members, articulated these traditional and contemporary concerns during her first interview: "I feel my body is ugly and I'm not really worthwhile! I realize I feel that most acutely after I speak to my parents. My father wants to know how the grades are. My mother asks, each time she calls, if I have put on weight. If I say yes, she tells me I won't be able to attract a man. Deep down inside I don't want to turn my back on my parents because I believe being skinny, an A student, and attracting a man with a desirable career will satisfy their demands as well as my own."

Many women who survive their adolescent years without disordered responses to food seem especially vulnerable during their early years at college. New opportunities present themselves, and new pressures move in. The experience of being a freshman, in somewhat threatening and unfamiliar surroundings, can be a traumatic one for even the most well adjusted young adult. The overprotected women we were seeing felt the separation from family most acutely. On their own for the first time in their lives, confronted by new people and possibilities, and away from the mealtime routines of the days when they lived at home, women who had never had weight problems began to put on pounds. Often family members reacted more negatively to the rapid weight gain than did the women themselves. One woman, who initially had satisfactory social experiences, had this to say: "Once in college I met guys right away and began to enjoy dating, and even kissing and making out as long as we didn't 'go too far.' Dates involved eating out a great deal—pizza and beer usually—and I returned home from this first year of college happy but 20 pounds heavier. At 5'2" and 125 pounds, I was pleasingly plump, but not to my mother, who was horrified with the changes in my body. My frequent snacking was looked on with disgust, so I was happy to return to college in the fall, away from my mother's disapproving eye."

When this young woman returned to college, she, like many others, shifted her dependency from family to the college itself. Campus life, although frightening, provided a certain structure and protection and a hope for the future. The women came to view college as "their big chance" (some viewed it as their last chance), and their definition of success was rigid and extreme: they must receive straight A's and they must be pursued by men. If they received lower marks than those to which they were accustomed, they felt despair. If they were not socially active and did not form intimate relationships with men, they considered themselves worthless and incomplete.

With such expectations, they set themselves up for failure. In the seventies, campuses had lost the freewheeling sense of camaraderie fostered by the political activism and defiance of the sixties. The academic atmosphere was more serious, and good grades harder to maintain. Noses were to the grindstone, competition was fierce, and students felt more isolated and lonely. The women's movement had made some inroads, but even if some women had acquired a new consciousness, it was clear that many more defined themselves in terms of male approval. If they were not sought after by men, they were failures.

The women we were seeing had a long history of perfectionism, and they were of above-average intelligence. For the most part, they had done well at school and felt somewhat secure in this area (although they were quick to characterize themselves as social failures). Thus, an increased push toward academic achievement quickly became their way of compensating for feelings of social inadequacy and self-doubt—especially if male attention was not immediately forthcoming. Eventually, however, even academic success failed to counter the emptiness they experienced when their expectations of being pursued by men did not materialize. As we have seen, the majority of these women had been both desirous of and frightened by male contact during adolescence. Now, feeling an intense urgency to form intimate relationships, they believed themselves unattractive, undesirable, and unworthy, and many turned to food for solace.

Some women spoke of food as an "inadequate means of coping, a return to old childhood security." For others, eating became a form of entertainment. "I was eating alone for the first time in my life." The change in eating habits was often bolstered by the fact that "others were in the same boat." One of our freshman coeds said: "The first eating bout that could be classified as a binge was during a period of loneliness when I felt overwhelmed by the size of Cornell. Heterosexual relationships were nil at this point and the only pressure I felt to be thin was the sign of thin girls and dieting friends."

During their college years, other women turn away from food and toward "the diet" in hopes of finding the key to social success. When their expectations for a magical transformation are not realized, they, like their adolescent counterparts, often begin to binge after one or several dieting attempts have failed. Initially, as in the following example, they may not have been overweight, but they then allow themselves to become a slave to "the habit": "At the beginning of my freshman year of college, I decided that at 128 pounds and 5'6", I was fat. I began a crash diet and lost 15 pounds. During the next summer I lived away from home by myself and literally ate myself into 160 pounds of ugliness out of loneliness. I began to purge out of total desperation soon after."

Thus, dieting characterized by extreme denial is often followed by binges that may continue for months. "During the summer between my freshman and sophomore years of college, I lost 35 pounds and continued to diet through Thanksgiving, being very proud of the fact that I made it through a Thanksgiving dinner with the family without cheating. Actually, in five months I had never once deviated from the diet I was following, never had even one bite of 'illegal' food. I came back to school after the holiday and went to dinner with some friends. I suddenly decided to have a piece of chocolate cream pie. Once I ate this, I felt there was nothing stopping me. I felt singularly directed— I had to have another 'bad' thing to eat. I went immediately to the store and bought a bag of cookies; next I had some ice cream and on and on. This binge didn't let up until February. Never once did I feel I had control over this process. I blamed the binge, the weight gain, my

depression, *everything,* on that one piece of pie. I said over
and over 'if only I hadn't eaten the pie.' It was as though I
had an ultimately fatal disease—although there were
periods of remission, it was certainly a terminal case with
no real hope of recovery."

Some women do experience moderate social success, but
not enough to give them the necessary confidence. Even
while they are dating, a chance remark about weight by a
man can precipitate the destructive eating pattern. Ellen
traces her problem to such an experience: "Early in my
sophomore year I met Peter, my future husband. He told
me, practically on our first date, that if I lost a little weight
I'd be beautiful. I began dieting strenuously at that point
and lost 25 pounds. I soon became compulsive about keeping my weight at 98 throughout my college years and did
so by replacing pizza and beer with yogurt, grapefruit and
black coffee." Although Ellen was able to maintain her
"ideal" weight throughout college, she gained a few pounds
when she was in graduate school. She tried a number of
dieting methods without success and then remembered that
a college roommate with a similar problem had forced herself to vomit. Ellen was so unhappy with her weight gain
that she tried this method. It seemed to work, so she began
an eight-year pattern of binge-ing and purging.

Those women who have already initiated a binge / purge
cycle in adolescence face additional obstacles to intimacy
with men once they enter college. The binge / purge cycle
of bulimarexics is so confining that an inordinate amount
of energy is expended simply in the behavior, and the
women are unable to concentrate on anything else. Paradoxically, these women who yearn so intensely for intimacy report feeling most vulnerable when they are with
men. They are then at their most isolated, living in a way

that is basically dishonest, and convinced that they must hide their inner selves from the world. They live in dread that their eating habits will be exposed and that men will reject them. Most of these women have had limited dating experience and therefore lack confidence in social situations.

Many of the women we treated had never had a lasting or loving relationship with a man. They hoped therapy would help them change in ways that would make "guys turn on." Success was defined as losing more weight and staying that way. Lacking any insight into their problem, they could not (would not) feel "whole" without a man. If only "Prince Charming" would appear, everything would be all right. At the same time, they were unable to see how their neediness and desperation drove men to reject them. These women have great difficulty viewing themselves as capable of developing into strong and independent women. In their encounters with men, they are constantly trying to find out what the man likes. If he is a tennis player, they take up tennis. If classical music is his interest, they follow that pursuit with a vengeance. A woman named Stephanie told us: "I knocked myself out doing things that were against my nature. All for the purpose of making him notice me. The relationship ended after a few months. My problems in concentration started soon after. He used to be my motivation all through school and then he dropped away. Schoolwork became meaningless. If I could have anything or anybody, I would still want him. I have a feeling only another man can take my mind off this preoccupation."

Another woman said: "I've been guiding my life toward my Prince Charming, and it's probably not going to happen. That's pretty scary."

Recently, we addressed the student body of a small eastern college about our research and treatment of bulimarexia. During the question-and-answer period, a coed mentioned a letter to the editor of their campus newspaper that had created a furor. The facts were a bit fuzzy, but evidently a male student had written to say that the women students of the college had "let themselves go" physically. He described them as having "fat asses." The coed cited the letter as an example of the ways men put women under pressure. During her presentation, Marlene had indicated that in spite of the so-called "new feminism," the present model of extreme slimness was being imposed *on women by women*, i. e., men do not prefer Twiggies! This woman was saying no to Marlene and using the letter to show that men expected extreme thinness in women. After the letter appeared in the newspaper, widespread dieting among the women resulted, and some began to dread eating in the dining centers. Not only were they convinced that male students were watching them eat, but they began to watch each other eat as well. As this woman was telling her story, we noticed many other women nodding in agreement. What was most significant and striking to us were the women's own reactions to the opinion of *one* man. Rather than ignoring the letter or responding with humor (even anger), these women believed themselves unattractive and, by extension, incapable of attracting men.

The ability to reward herself, to feel her own self-worth, is foreign to the bulimarexic, who seems intent on pleasing others and being perfect. Ironically, her very behavior serves to keep her socially isolated. Anne's story provides a fairly typical example. For months, Anne had been secretly fasting and binge-ing. Then she was invited out to dinner by a young man with whom she was infatuated. She wanted to accept the date, but was in the fasting part of her cycle. She was afraid that she would give in to temptation and eat and thus worked herself into a high state of anxiety. Should she go on the date or stay at home? She did accept, ate moderately at dinner, and had an enjoyable time. But after the man had seen her home, the stress of the evening proved to be too much for her, and she began to binge grotesquely. The disgust that followed her binge provided Anne with an excuse to withdraw from further social encounters.

Many women like Anne are so frightened by the possibility of rejection that it seems safer to hide behind fat or disgust than to risk actual engagement. Because of their low self-esteem, these women feel unworthy of being loved and can attribute this feeling to their temporary self-disgust about binge-ing or being slightly overweight. Binge-ing wards off people with a "wall of (perceived) fat." It is a way of "filling up" without needing others.

The woman so afflicted becomes locked into a struggle between two parts of herself. Total control versus being out of control—being "good" versus being "bad." The bulimarexic, believing herself unlovable, then becomes supersensitive to the reactions of others. The most minor or insignificant slight is exaggerated and distorted, creating massive self-loathing that propels the woman to further binge-ing. The anger she feels toward her imagined "rejector" is not acknowledged. Instead, it is turned inward, adding to the fury of the binge.

The insidious fear of rejection often evolves into irrational and crippling thoughts. These naïve and unassertive women focus on rejection alone, rather than on the man who has rejected them. They rarely examine his human failings, nor can they conceive of themselves as fortunate to be rid of someone who does not value them. There is a "life and death" quality to these relationships even when it is clear that the women are only marginally involved. It does not seem to matter if they do not even *like* the man who has rejected them or if the man has obviously been using and / or abusing them. Being rejected therefore is equated with being a "failure." Significantly, most lack the courage to ask their partners about what went wrong. They weave a rich fantasy around the experience, assuming the worst—that they have been rejected because they are too fat!

Some bulimarexic women do develop intimate relationships with men. This can lead to a "remission" of symptoms (as long as these caring men are in the picture). Once involved with a man, however, they typically rechannel most of the energy they have been expending on bingeing and purging into a mutually destructive / dependent relationship. Aimee Liu, the author of *Solitaire,* appears deliberately to have made this trade off when she chose to apply to the same college her boyfriend was attending: "It suddenly occurred to me that love might help me escape the tyranny of my eating compulsions, that in fact those compulsions were probably offshoots of loneliness and insecurity. All the stuffing and subsequent self-abuse had helped to pass time that should have been devoted to someone else. But now that Ken was ready to save me, I could normalize."

Rather than residing in a college dorm, Aimee moved in with her boyfriend and did in fact "normalize" her eating behavior. Hovever, she soon found that she had become an extension of Ken. Eventually, she had to break this dependency before she could grow as a healthy and self-actualized woman.

Such relationships, while relieving the surface of the bulimarexic's problem, are generally ultimately destructive. The neediness of these women makes the possibility of success uncertain, and termination of the affair is experienced as devastating—driving the woman even deeper into hopelessness and helplessness, and increasing her anger toward men.

Some, while in the throes of such relationships, resume their binge-ing, thereby resorting to dishonesty and subterfuge. Even if they are competent in all other aspects of their lives, they do not feel whole, functioning, or "normal." They live in fear that they will be "found out." Since these women have invested their men with heroic qualities, they can only experience themselves as smaller and weaker by comparison. Believing themselves so unworthy, they are grateful that women as "screwed up" and disgusting as themselves could be lucky encough to find men who love them. Since they also believe that their men "love a lie," they necessarily experience themselves as "phony" and unreal.

Heterosexual relationships then are a parody—an exaggeration of all that is wrong with these women's lives. However powerless and helpless they may feel in relation to school or family, they are even more debilitated when involved in relationships that are sexual. Sexuality is a great wasteland of unfulfilled pleasures, confusion, guilt, fear, and disgust. For these are protected and relatively innocent women who have generally been brought up to be "good girls." Promiscuity, liberal or carefree sexual attitudes, and multiple sexual relationships are conspicuously absent from their lives. The following is a typical comment: "I have always been very naïve about sexual relationships. I can remember pondering whether it was a sin when someone touched my breast for the first time when I was nineteen! I was shocked to learn that my roommate had been sleeping with her boyfriend since she was sixteen."

Our research suggests that sex and sexual fantasies play an important part in the lives of these women. Here we are not referring to the fantasy of oral impregnation that appears in much of the analytic literature about women with eating disorders, but to the fear of rejection by the sexual partner. In other words, the woman is afraid she is not "good enough" to please a man. Bulimarexics are, of course, not alone in these fears. Most women have been conditioned to accept men as more experienced sexually and to expect them to be the teachers in sexual matters.

In addition, the lifetime socialization of women trains them to derive their pleasure from *giving* rather from receiving. Until recently, the standards for appropriate sexual behavior have been set for women by men. Women should be supremely sensitive to the needs of the men they are involved with, always concerned that the men be satisfied. This preoccupation with pleasing men leads women to lose connection with their own desires and needs. Many bulimarexic women unquestioningly accept their partners' idea of what sexual activity is acceptable. When the women do not achieve satisfaction, they blame themselves, feel that they are failures. It seldom occurs to them to expect pleasure for its own sake (their pleasure is in giving), nor are they assertive enough or candid enough to indicate the kind of touching they find pleasurable. Thus, while many of these women are sexually active, they do not experience fulfillment. They feel they must go through whatever charade is necessary to secure the love and attention of their men. Some fake orgasm, while others seek to avoid sexual intercourse, though they may find kissing and caressing pleasurable, because they feel that intercourse leaves them vulnerable to rejection if their performance should not be considered satisfactory. Being a good sex partner is equated with being a "real woman."

Sometimes the fear of sexuality takes a different form. There are women who are afraid that their appetite for sex will become as insatiable as their appetite for food. Since they overwhelmingly feel out of control with regard to food, they come to feel that they are powerless over their sexual behavior as well. Consequently, they "binge on sex" on occasion and punish themselves with the same feelings of shame and self-disgust that they use against themselves after food orgies. Not surprisingly, such empty and dehumanizing sexual encounters often create a further stimulus for grotesque food binges. "I habitually use food as an insulator," one woman told us. "It protects me from sexual contact and promiscuity. When I am thin, I become sexual, constantly worrying about sexual performance and wondering if I will be able to have an orgasm this time. Wondering if the man will know I feign it. Ironically, the men with whom I sleep invariably shower me with praise for my skill as a lover. Afterward I try to relieve my insecurity with food. After a man leaves my apartment, I rush to the mirror to see if yet another sexual encounter has changed me. It hasn't, so I will devote an entire day to binge-ing."

Along with the fear of being an inadequate sexual partner, bulimarexics typically loathe their bodies. They are certain that they will be rejected because they are too fat, and they believe that men will be horrified to see them undressed. If they do appear naked, they are likely to require constant reassurance that their bodies are attractive. Many allow themselves to sleep only in one position (on their stomachs), for fear that their lovers will see a protruding stomach. Such narcissistic self-absorption can cause their worst fears to come true. The lover who is badgered incessantly by the woman who asks if he thinks she's too fat is bound eventually to respond with anger or boredom.

Although recent research has indicated that men are more attracted to women's faces than to their bodies, bulimarexics think they already know what men really want. They are absolutely convinced that their bodies are imperfect; therefore, it is irrelevant what their men say to them.

Undoubtedly, Jackie, the woman whose story follows, would like to be thought of as a sharp lady who is exciting to be with, but her preoccupation with appearance has narrowed her to the point where she is no longer stimulating or interesting. She may feel a perverse satisfaction that her lover has confirmed her deepest fears, and she may not realize that she is the one who is driving him away. Jackie and women like her turn themselves into sexual objects, albeit unwittingly. Often, the men with whom they have relationships want women who are quite different from the image the bulimarexics hold in mind. This man, Jackie's fiance, at his wit's end, wrote the following: "Lately, all our conversations center around Jackie's body. She used to be witty, fun, and exciting. I was attracted to her enthusiasm and her mind. She was and still is (although I'm beginning to doubt this) a very sharp lady. However, she now sounds like a broken record. After we finish talking about her body she has nothing to say. I could care less if she's ten to fifteen pounds heavier and that is the God's honest truth! In fact, I would prefer it, as right now she looks like a Cambodian refugee! Of course, though, she doesn't believe me. She insists she knows *what I really like*—even what I am thinking. I find this infuriating."

Few bulimarexics report that they started binge-ing and purging while married, although several turn to this form of solace when separated or divorced. Many, however, vow to give up gorging and purging once they are married. The hope is that marriage itself will magically transform their lives. For some, this does happen, and they experience long remissions. Others resume their habit in secret, feeling more guilty and ashamed than ever. And with good reason, for their lives are filled with further subterfuge. Now, in addition to binge-ing and purging, the woman depletes her engery with games she must invent to "cover her tracks." She has little time for anything other than nurturing the behavior, engaging in it, and hiding it. Honesty, intimacy, and mutual respect become impossible under such circumstances. When these marriages fail, the men may never really know what happened. Unbelievable as it may seem, bulimarexics have managed to keep their behavior a total secret from husbands and other loved ones for as long as ten to fifteen years. Upon observing their wives' exaggerated sense of privacy, some husbands suspect the worst: "She must be having an affair," they conclude. If their wives do reveal a "problem with food," these husbands are vastly relieved; a food problem seems insignificant when compared to what they had fantasized. Other husbands are bewildered by what they see as abuse of the body. From boyhood, they have been taught to "build up" and conserve their bodies, not to tear them down, and they have always viewed themselves as *much more* than their bodies alone. As Susan Sontag pointed out in her article "The Double Standard of Aging," men are conditioned to feel that it is not masculine to care so much about their looks (while women are conditioned "to care too much"). Thus, many men, no matter how sympathetic they might be, find the excessive vanity of bulimarexics ludicrous, frivolous, foolish, and downright boring. They honestly cannot comprehend that women could make themselves slaves to food. In their confusion, they deny that there is a problem and somehow believe that if they ignore it, it will go away. When wives finally reach out for help from these men, the response is often totally unexpected: "His reaction was very similar to what many people had said to me. Psychiatrists, for instance. What I told him went in one ear and out the other. I couldn't convey the intensity of my problem to him. My food binges didn't seem like a serious thing—he thought I was ridiculous."

One woman who had maintained bulimarexia through-out twelve years of marriage finally chose her thirteenth wedding anniversary as the time to "confess." Her husband responded with a burst of laughter and refused to listen to her further attempts to explain. In so doing, he was giving her an all clear to continue the binge / purge behavior because the message implicit in his reaction was "It's not so serious" or "It's okay for you to do this screwy thing." In this case, revealing the secret created further conflict as communication was still blocked. Husbands can also use the confession as leverage with their wives, controlling them through threats of exposure or rejection. Furthermore, with this new ammunition they can retaliate if their wives dare to criticize them for their own imperfections.

Other husbands become suspicious and angry. Not knowing what course to take, they adopt a "watchdog" stance, which often makes matters worse. One despairing husband put it this way: "This problem controls her whole schedule and dictates that much time be devoted to her problem. She cheats both herself and me out of time. I feel she lies to "cover" her secret behaviour. She locks bathroom doors so she can engage in her habit in privacy, and then I start assuming she's engaging in binge-ing or more likely vomiting, especially when this occurs after I go to bed."

Husbands who refuse to take bulimarexia seriously are not necessarily insensitive or uncaring. Some are initially understanding, but when the behavior does not lessen, they reach their limits. Typically, they say they do not care if their wives are slightly overweight—they just want them to be happy again, the way they were at some earlier time. Afraid for the future, these men are actually trying to encourage their wives to be stronger and less dependent. Intuitively, they feel that they are lending support to the behavior if they monitor their wives or become too involved in their care. They want to see their wives take more responsibility for their own actions, to see them be *partners* in the truest sense, and they are motivated by love and an understanding of contemporary psychology. The dangerous nature of too much involvement is clearly illustrated by a conversation we had with a demoralized husband a few years ago. This man called one evening and insisted on speaking to Bill. In desperation, he wanted to know if he was doing the right thing. For the last few months, his wife had asked him to assist her in throwing up after binge-ing by standing behind her and pulling on her stomach. She said she could not vomit by herself. This man loved his wife, but obviously felt deeply uncertain about her request. Bill simply asked him how he felt about *his* participation in the ritual. Apparently, the man had seldom been asked about *his* feelings. He said he was disgusted by what he was doing. In fact, he knew that his wife's binges had increased since he took on the role of accomplice. Bill told him that it was appropriate for him to feel such revulsion, and this seemed to help. The man told his wife that he honestly felt she was killing herself and their relationship and that he could not aid and abet her any longer. He insisted that she seek treatment immediately. After some resistance, she did.

What is going wrong in these marriages? For the most part, bulimarexics trade their individual talents and outside activities for the romantic ideal of security, safety, and living happily ever after with their husbands. Eagerly discarding career objectives in order to devote themselves to the wife / homemaker role, they now have feelings of "entitlement." In return, they should be rescued from responsibility and cared for. However, *vicarious* living is especially difficult for bulimarexics since before marriage they were generally high achievers. The burden for bulimarexics is their *history*. Most, at one point or another, have been rewarded for their accomplishments and have experienced the exhilaration of using their talents. It is an experience they yearn for again and again, even though they have locked themselves into a limited role.

Current research indicates that level of education is an important variable in marriage satisfaction. According to many surveys, college educated women are consistently less satisfied with the homemaker role than those without such an education. With fewer sources of outside gratification available, they soon become bored, depressed, and unhappy. In time, a husband's successes coupled with the wife's increasing emptiness and envy often signify the death of a marriage. Shirley, college-educated and a talented musician, is a good example. Her family and friends were overjoyed when she met, captured, and married Sam, a well-known surgeon. Sad to say, her own years of accomplishment as a concert pianist had never elicited as much acceptance and excitement. After three years of comparative idleness, Shirley, feeling herself an extension of Sam, began to have minor but unpredictable temper tantrums. In reaction, Sam began to spend more and more time at the hospital. Shirley, in a panic at losing Sam, alternated between "total woman" tactics and withdrawal. Since Shirley had given up bulimarexia "forever" on the day she married, this obviously was not her problem *now*. However, she almost wished it were because she was unable, even with the help of intensive psychotherapy, to understand what her real conflicts were. She believed, and therapy reinforced the belief, that she had everything she had ever dreamed of. So what was wrong with her. Why couldn't she relax, and be nice, appreciative, and grateful? What Shirley thought she "should" feel prevented her from ever facing up to her lack of fulfillment in a direct fashion. In part, this was not Shirley's fault. Like many women, she had chosen a man whose credentials were "perfect." By comparison, Shirley felt inadequate and insignificant, and since she had abandoned her concert career without a backward glance, it was hard for Sam to take her talent seriously. She, in turn, reinforced this by "playing for Sam" (i.e., popular music), thus giving up playing what she loved most—Beethoven and Bach. Eventually, Sam grew tired of Shirley's instability and nagging and walked out. On that day she resumed the old familiar habit she had given up four years before—binge-ing and purging.

Colette Dowling, in *The Cinderella Complex: Women's Hidden Fear of Independence,* captures some of the dynamics of bulimarexic women when she describes the way in which married women embrace drudge work to preserve their illusion of security and to avoid challenging responsibilities as well as their terror of aloneness and the unknown. Dowling's book is about the ways women themselves contribute to their own states of helplessness and nurture the desire to merge with another person. The book is provocative because Dowling exposes the ways women manipulate and exploit men in order to get them to take care of them so that they can lead childlike, easy, and unchallenged lives.

In our group therapy program, many married bulimarexic women have concluded that this behavior is characteristic of them. By relinquishing responsibility and embracing the role of the "sick one," the bulimarexic creates further conflicts for her husband as well as for herself. Anne's husband Paul, a concerned and loving man, felt at least partially responsible for her unhappiness. She felt he loved his work more than her, and Paul, out of a genuine desire to help Anne through her "crisis," began to spend more time at home. Anne had literally taken to bed after being laid off from a high status job. The state of the economy rather than poor performance had resulted in the layoff, but Anne had chosen to do nothing and had become very depressed. She returned to a childhood pattern of overeating, gained fifteen pounds in only six weeks, and then refused to go out. Although she had often gained weight and then fasted during similar stress periods while in college, she had triumphantly stablilized her eating habits for the two years of her marriage. As his worries increased, Paul began giving up those physical activities he used to let off steam after a grueling day as a salesman. He stopped playing squash with his buddies and gave up his greatest love—fly-fishing in the wilderness. His role as caretaker for Anne only seemed to make matters worse. When he complied with Anne's requests to keep her from eating by locking cabinets, she became angry, even defiant, and accused him of "not really wanting to be with her." In fact, her accusation was starting to become a reality. She was becoming harder and harder to love. Paul felt he was "the man," the one who should be able to solve the problem. However, lately he had been feeling more and more ineffectual.

Numerous concerned men have shared similar feelings of despair and frustration over "losing their wives," women who have obviously expected more from them than any one person could provide. The pain and victimization of these men is as intense as that of their partners.

Of course, there are husbands whose personal problems are overwhelming. Many bulimarexics simply have terrible marital relationships that can hardly be considered the end result of bulimarexia, although it might be said that their fantasies of rescue kept them from seeing men clearly in the first place. Whether the men are alcoholic, irresponsible, self-occupied, or downright hostile and abusive, a terrifying fear of "being alone" combined with a paralyzing sense of guilt and helplessness keeps the women imprisoned in destructive relationships with them. Most of these women have been conditioned to believe it is up to them to make the marriage work, even when there is no longer anything to be retrieved. There must be something they are doing wrong or should be doing right. They suffer all kinds of abuse as the price for holding onto the illusion that things will get better if they just try harder, or love more, or seek therapy. For these desperately unhappy women, gorging and purging can become a crucial coping mechanism. Their marriages will continue to be terrible whether or not they give up the behavior. Binge-ing and purging serves to keep the painful reality of their lives temporarily buried. Instead of making a decision—in short, taking action—they prefer treading water, avoiding, and hoping.

Some bulimarexic women do attempt to break away from mutually destructive marriages. Unfortunately, many act impulsively. They may abruptly move out of the house, hoping that they will be able to give up bulimarexia. After all, most continue to believe that bulimarexia is their real problem, not their husbands or their marriages. If they can just resolve their food problem everything will be OK! But now they are alone with their food. Almost invariably, they crash and return home to their husbands. Those who manage to make the break from their marital relationships generally transfer their dependency needs back to families, friends, or therapists. With few supports available, they are unable to move forward on their own. In a particularly poignant letter, one woman stated: "I had reached the point where I was having trouble coping with day-to-day activities. I couldn't get out of bed and go to work. I was really in bad shape, and I wasn't able to confide in my husband, get help from him. I didn't have any friends where we were. I called my family out of desperation, not knowing what to do. I just cried . . . didn't really tell them what was going on. Just told them eveything was terrible, and my father said, 'Come home. We'll take care of you. We'll make everything better.' " And so this woman traded one kind of dependency for another more benign form.

What if there are children? Does the prospect of caring for another human being who is even more helpless and dependent cause a change in behavior? Once again, the expectations of many bulimarexic women are unrealistic. There is always the hope that an outside situation will release them magically from their disordered eating behavior. And, in most cases, they experience disappointment. As one woman told us: "I can recall only one week of abstinence after my pregnancy. I was afraid that vomiting would tear my stitches. You see, even the fear that I might hurt my unborn child would not make me stop this habit."

Bulimarexic women who continue their behavior throughout childbirth and the rearing of children often seem more helpless and desperate than their married, childless counterparts. For, in addition to feelings of shame and self-disgust, they carry the added burden of believing that they are "bad mothers." Their guilt is often overwhelming.

Many mothers report that they looked forward to childbirth, believing their eating compulsion would be replaced with new goals and self-fulfilling activities. In addition to child care, some become compulsive house cleaners or harness their own compulsion to eat by becoming gourmet cooks for others—children, husbands, and friends. They throw themselves into a frenzy of activity that makes them seem the perfect mother and wife. More than likely, however, these women resume their habitual binge-ing patterns: "I don't want to die, but I am killing myself. I have two children and yet my obsession with food comes first. I work and cook a decent meal for my children every night, which I don't eat. I wait until they are through, eat everything they haven't, which is usually a lot, and then eat everything else I can find, usually sweet. I am a good mother, *I guess,* but I hate myself."

Still living through others, they are essentially the same

passive, dependent, and nonassertive women they were at the time they married. While family responsibilities and society's expectations have broadened and become more complex, their inner selves are still embryonic, fuzzy, and undefined.

Bulimarexic wives and mothers often point wistfully to the unmarried, career women in our groups. Most are amazed that these supposedly independent women also feel dissatisfaction and emptiness. They find it confusing, for our therapy emphasizes the need for more than one identity and for taking action and risks. Here are these attractive and talented women, out in the world and growing through their success. But are they? The fact is that more than a few of these professional women envy the married woman. They would gladly set aside the anxiety involved in daily risk taking and confrontation for the comfort and security they believe is inherent in marriage and childbearing. Some even express resentment that *they have to* support themselves. Unlike married bulimarexics, single career women do not usually binge out of boredom. On the contrary, their lives are often *too* full, and as perpetual people pleasers they habitually take on more than they can handle. Their binge-ing is often precipitated because of their unwillingness to say no and give themselves a break. Becoming a career woman does not signal the death of the "good girl." In spite of their achievements, many still have great difficulty dealing with disapproval and criticism. Besides, now that they have proven their success to all, there is constant pressure to continue doing so. Thus, it is not surprising that few of our professional women are comfortable with the power associated with the work world or with the excellence that is now expected of them.

Of course, we have encountered professional women

who do gain real satisfaction from their careers and they have every intention of continuing to work, whether or not they become wives and mothers. Their hope is that they will be able to combine all the roles. Their problem lies not in career overinvolvement but in social underinvolvement. They may have professional strengths, but they are still shy and nonassertive with men. They long for heterosexual relationships but lack confidence and social skills. In one very important way, they are similar to married bulimarexics—they continue to value the importance of relationships with men above all else and to give men the power to define how they should act, think, and feel.

CHAPTER 6

Bulimarexia and the Body

Our aim in this chapter is not to "scare" women out of binge-ing and purging. Scare tactics are seldom successful in convincing people to change habits, and the cyclical eating pattern of bulimarexics is unusually well entrenched. However, we do want to make women aware of the damage they may be inflicting on their bodies. The physiological ramifications of the binge and purge have received scant professional attention, so more research is necessary before this aspect of bulimarexia can be fully understood. The factual material presented here is simply a beginning. It includes what we have learned from medical colleagues and the literature. We have also drawn extensively on what we have learned from bulimarexic clients—among them women who are physicians, nurses, and nutritionists.

If some women are persuaded, after reading this chapter, to modify their binge / purge behavior, we would be enormously pleased. Equally important, if we can motivate them to speak directly and candidly to their physicians—revealing all aspects of their problem—we will feel justified in outlining some alarming findings that have yet to be endorsed by the medical community. Only if women speak out can they be truly helped. At the same time, we hope that by focusing attention on what we consider a major threat to women's health, we can help professionals to question and examine their patients more thoroughly. For, as we have pointed out repeatedly, the bulimarexic's covert pleas for help are usually overlooked or misinterpreted.

THE BINGE

Binge-eating is well recognized as a problem among people of all weight levels. Independent research at Duke and Stanford Universities has indicated that approximately 50 percent of the obese patients surveyed binged on large quantities of food at least once a week.

Our survey data with regard to bulimarexics is even more dramatic. Of 300 bulimarexics recently surveyed, 82 percent indicated that they binged at least three times a week.

Bingers tend to prefer high calorie "junk food," although they will binge on anything that is readily available. Fast foods, high in sugar content, which require little preparation are prime binge foods, particularly when they can be quickly purchased and consumed in private. Here are some of the problems that can result.

Hypoglycemia

Many bulimarexics attribute their dizziness, headaches, fatigue, numbness, irritability, crying, excessive worry, anxiety, and depression to a syndrome known as hypoglycemia. Hypoglycemia literally refers to a deficiency of sugar

in the blood. Although it is at the opposite pole from dia-
betes, it can paradoxically lead to that disease. In hypoglycemia, the body, in response to foods high in sugar
content, triggers the pancreas to release an excess of insulin. This drives blood sugar levels below normal, often creating a craving for *more* sugar—the very substance that
initiated the disorder in the first place. Thus, hypoglyce-
mics often turn to the very foods that are forbidden them
in order to satisfy this "craving." Examples of these "forbidden foods" are sugar, honey, pizza, breads made from
refined white flour, potatoes, corn, rice, and sugar-
sweetened soft drinks.

In the mid-1970s, Drs. Cheraskin and Ringsdorf of the
University of Alabama's Department of Oral Medicine
drew attention to an alarming increase in the incidence of
hypoglycemia, and they identified changing technology as
the culprit. Specifically, it was their contention that hor-
monal deficiencies and lack of trace minerals that are
essential to sugar metabolism were caused by the improper
milling of flour and refinement of sugar—practices that
grew out of our twentieth-century obsession with white-
ness in flour and sugar. Crucial vitamins, minerals, and
amino acids were thereby being eliminated from the average diet, according to these researchers. As a result of this
hypothesis, many a bulimarexic embraced hypoglycemia
as her cause celebré.

Recently, other researchers who may have been more
attuned to the binge / purge practices of thousands of
women began to question this "craving for sugar" excuse
of the bulimarexic. Dr. L. M. Vincent, writing in *Competing
with the Sylph,* feels that the incidence of true chemical
hypoglycemia has been exaggerated, often serving as a
convenient "whipping boy" for those women who fail to

acknowledge or are unaware of the harm they are causing their bodies by gorging and purging. Dr. Vincent indicates that a combination of psychological and physiological factors contribute to the desire to binge, i.e., severe carbohydrate restriction could lead to carbohydrate craving. Under such circumstances, it is dangerous for the chronic binger to hide behind the hypoglycemic label, for in so doing she not only finds an excuse for her inability to maintain proper nutrition, but subbornly refuses to explore alternative sources of her problem. She has a disease and, as with all good patients, she must be cured (by someone else!).

Dr. Vincent therefore emphasizes the importance of distinguishing "pseudohypoglycemia," which can be traced to the poor nutritional status of the binge / purger, from true, chemical hypoglycemia.

Anecdotal evidence gleaned from the bulimarexics we have treated supports the view that poor diet and stress initiate the fatigue, dizziness, and anxiety associated with pseudohypoglycemia. These symptoms have usually been reversible within a few months and bulimarexics who embark on appropriate corrective nutritional programs report being considered healthy soon again by their internists. Initiation and maintenance of this supplemental medical treatment was, however, in *every* case related to the woman's willingness to enter psychotherapy and honestly confront the problem on more than one level. For this reason, we have developed a referral network of informed internists, endocrinologists, and nutritionists who are prepared to aid the bulimarexic who is determined to help herself. Such an interdisciplinary approach should be an integral part of any comprehensive treatment program.

Metabolic Considerations

Bulimarexics apparently do not realize that fat synthesis and accumulation are necessary for survival. Fat is the main storage form of body energy, although sugar, stored in our muscles, is our most efficient energy source. However, sugar is in limited supply and when it is depleted, fatigue and exhaustion ultimately occur. Thus, under the usual demands of our daily routine, we first draw upon fatty acids (fat) as a major source of energy. In fact, doctors tell us that with mild exercise, fat contributes twice as much energy as does sugar. However, when fat levels are depleted, the body must draw upon carbohydrates (sugar). Blood sugar level is therefore critical and is indirectly regulated by the pancreas, which releases insulin according to body needs. When we are hungry, as after exercise, sugar supplies dwindle so that insulin production stimulates the release of more sugar from body stores. The liver is the manufacturer of sugar; with fasting or exercise, it steps up its output. Studies of prolonged fasting show that body metabolism decreases and more energy is drawn from fat deposits in order to conserve valuable protein and water. Thus, the body functions adaptively under food deprivation in an attempt to get the most out of its available energy sources. The bulimarexic, in her chronic binge / purge ritual, often creates such "energy crises." Physicians with whom we have collaborated consistently express concern over the serious depletion of the bulimarexic's energy reserves. As a result of this depletion, the metabolic rate may decrease so that voluntary lethargy can ensue. Such a state of mind will, in time, foster pessimism and inactivity, common precursors to a major problem among bulimarexics—depression.

Psychotrophic Drugs

Bulimarexics who seek help are occasionally taking drugs that are classified as "psychotrophic"; that is, they effect psychic functioning and / or experience. Among them are the phenothiazine derivatives (Compazine, Phenergan, Stelazine, Temeral, Thorazine) and the tricyclic antidepressants (Elavil, Nardil, Tofranil, and Triavil, to mention a few of the better known). Because such drugs are known to influence food craving and enhance binge-ing, they are capable of mimicking the kind of binge-eating associated with bulimarexia.

Furthermore, certain medications, if administered to bulimarexics (especially chronic vomiters), can result in death. Recently, a twenty-three-year-old nursing student, a chronic vomiter, was given Lithium while participating in a sleep research study conducted by the National Institute of Health. During screening, this young woman failed to reveal that she engaged in binge-vomiting and that it had involved her in two distinct bouts of cardiac arrest and an ensuing two-day coma. In general, Lithium depletes cells of potassium. This side effect presents no problem among those who eat regularly and do not vomit. However, in the case of this chronic vomiter, the loss of stomach acid apparently led to a compensatory loss of intracellular potassium, which doctors believe resulted in cardiac arrest and her death. Lithium should, therefore, never be administered to bulimarexics, especially to those who binge and vomit. Such findings are particularly relevant to the binger and her nonmedical therapist and serve to underline the tremendous risk inherent in the treatment process. It is therefore imperative that physicians be consulted and counseled regularly regarding the treatment of women engaged in this pernicious behavior.

Neurological Abnormalities

Recently, researchers have reported abnormalities in the electroencephalograms (EEGs) of certain bingers of varied weights. Dr. Albert Stunkard and his colleagues at the University of Pennsylvania are currently evaluating the impact of the drug Dilantin on certain bingers who appear to have specific subcortical dysregulation problems. Although initially encouraging, this important pilot work is not yet conclusive and the mechanism of action of this drug as well as the significance and prevalence of the neurological abnormalities remain uncertain. Nevertheless, these findings merit careful attention and the practitioner engaged in treating the bulimarexic should stay abreast of this work.

Psychological Factors

Finally, there are a number of aversive consequences of binge-ing that occur *after* the binge. Primary among these are anxiety and depression (created by astronomical food bills, lying, stealing, and hiding) as well as severe stomach pains, headaches, and dizziness. These bodily sensations, painful in their own right, often lead to serious accidents. For example, Liz, after gorging on junk food one evening, experienced violent abdominal cramping, a severe headache, and, in a frantic attempt to get back to her apartment, fell in front of a car, sustaining multiple fractures and a life-threatening concussion!

Bulimarexics tend to inflict severe self-criticism, resentment, and other forms of punishment upon themselves after binge-ing. Depressive episodes are not uncommon, often serving to motivate the woman to seek help. In fact, reexamination of the records of over one hundred and fifty women who we ultimately treated for bulimarexia revealed that over 40 percent of them had sought therapy earlier for depression. Of all the consequences of binge-ing, depression may well prove to be the most frequent and debilitating. We encounter more and more women who in desperation make suicide gestures and attempts. More often than not these depressive episodes are associated with the binge / purge ritual.

THE PURGE

Purging, by whatever means, becomes ritualized and tenacious. Bulimarexics report that purgative methods become relatively effortless as time goes on, so that the purges increase in frequency, intensity, and duration. Purging appears to be more deleterious physiologically than binge-ing, although binge-ing inevitably sets the stage for purging and, as such, assumes the central role. There are those who assert that if binge-ing can be eliminated, purging will no longer occur. This is simply not the case. In fact, several of our clients report that they rarely over-ate (by anyone's standards), yet they purged routinely after consuming modest amounts of food. The purge had been adopted as the most "effective" way to prevent weight gain.

Most bulimarexic women have at one time or another stopped purging; yet they continue to overeat or binge uncontrollably due to their basic fear of becoming fat—a fear that will obviously not be curbed merely by eliminating purging. If the bulimarexic is to free herself from her disorder completely and permanently, she must be prepared to relinquish *both* habits and learn to fortify herself with new, more adaptive, habits that satisfy those same needs that maintained her cyclical ritual.

Self-induced Vomiting

Among the 300 bulimarexics we recently interviewed, the frequency of purging by self-induced vomiting varied from once weekly to eighteen times per day. Those who had vomited daily for five or more years often indicated that they suffered from reverse peristalsis, a condition involving spontaneous regurgitation of the stomach contents. This uncontrollable, painful behavior serves to stimulate more frequent purging so that many felt they had trouble keeping any food down for more than a few minutes.

According to a recent study by Jill Carni, a Boston psychotherapist who specializes in eating disorders, published in the *Journal of the Massachusetts Dental Society,* chronic vomiting can erode dental enamel, particularly on the inner surface of the teeth, due to the hydrochloric acid content of vomit. This erosion can be compounded by a diet limited to citrus fruits and may also result in severe gum disease, innumerable cavities, and tooth loss, which is also augmented by the heightened sugar intake and poor nutritional habits so common among bulimarexics.

Vomiting has also led to severe tearing and bleeding in and around the esophagus (throat). Hiatal hernias (the stomach pushing through the diaphragm, which creates the sensation of choking) and severely infected salivary glands are also commonly reported. One dental hygienist indicated that twenty of her patients, *all* of whom were women, had been forced eventually to undergo salivary or parotid gland surgery. Thus, the dentist, not the physician or psychotherapist, may be the first to encounter the ramifications of bulimarexic behavior.

Hypokalemia

The poor nutrition and restricted salt and mineral intake that often accompany chronic vomiting may result in a deficiency state referred to as hypokalemia (potassium deficiency). Postassium is necessary for adequate muscle functioning, and a deficiency is often marked by muscle fatigue, weakness, numbness, erratic heart beat, kidney damage, and, in severe instances, paralysis. Low levels of potassium can be brought about by chronic vomiting or diuretic abuse. The loss of potassium-containing foods and stomach acids by vomiting serves to precipitate additional imbalances that, in extreme cases, involve sodium and severe dehydration. These deficiency states can require immediate medical intervention. A nationally known athlete recently referred to us by her internist had fainted during an important competition after chronic self-induced vomiting had drastically lowered her potassium level. Despite this life threatening experience, she had withheld critical information from her physician. It was not until she entered the group that she admitted the severity and duration of her purging behavior!

Kidney problems are another probable consequence of an electrolyte imbalance. In 1979 *Psychological Medicine* published an article by Dr. Gerald Russell of the Department of Psychiatry, Royal Free Hospital, London, describing a patient suffering from what Russell refers to as "bulimia nervosa" (his term for bulimarexia), who developed kidney failure and hypertension after eight years of self-induced vomiting. A kidney transplant was ultimately required, and, upon recovery, the patient still resorted to occasional bouts of vomiting. Epileptic-like seizure patterns as well as extreme muscle tetany (spasm) were also noted among some of his patients with extreme electrolyte imbalances.

Laxative and Diuretic Abuse

The use of laxatives or diuretics as a way of purging seems to be more frequent now than even five years ago. Our survey indicated that in 1978, the majority of bulimarexics (83 percent) were vomiters; however, by 1980, less than 68 percent relied on self-induced vomiting as a means of purging. Laxative and diuretic purges were considered easier to conceal and, in most instances, less painful than chronic vomiting.

Laxatives such as castor oil serve to liquify feces and act as irritants that increase peristalsis (movemement of the intestines). By so doing, they retard the action of the intestines in absorbing fluids or may actually prevent them from doing so. Epsom salts, on the other hand, tend to increase volume within the intestines by attracting water so that the gut swells. As a result, food is more rapidly eliminated. Mineral oils lubricate and thereby prevent fecal water from being reabsorbed as it passes through the intestines.

Diuretics (water pills) serve to rid the body of water and, if taken in amounts that exceed recommended dosage, can precipitate or enhance dehydration. During the premenstrual period when the level of estrogen is relatively high, women generally gain weight. (This weight gain is attributable to edema and is characterized by puffiness, particularly around the face and feet.) Diuretics are often used as a means of stimulating urination in order to relieve this swelling. If women experience considerable discomfort, diuretics may be prescribed by a physician. Bulimarexics admit that doctors often dispense diuretics when they purposely exaggerate their symptoms in order to prevent weight gain. In their attempts to get rid of the puffiness, these women often become dehydrated. In response, the kidneys reduce the amount of water and salt excreted from the body. Dehydration resulting from restricted food intake and chronic diuretic abuse often leads to a deficiency of sodium and potassium, which in turn creates an electrolyte imbalance. Under these circumstances, the kidneys prefer to retain sodium at the expense of potassium, which is slowly excreted. The final result is muscle weakness, numbness, and, ultimately, paralysis.

Dehydration and electrolyte imbalances due to enhanced potassium loss through the gastrointestinal tract can also result from prolonged laxative abuse. Chronic abusers typically suffer severe constipation, due to the loss of intestinal muscle tone, and become more and more dependent upon laxatives. An alarming number of laxative abusers have acknowledged that they must consume over fifty laxatives daily in their attempt to maintain bowel control! Furthermore, abuse of irritant laxatives (e.g., castor oil, cascara) over a period of years can produce severe intestinal abnormalities that simulate inflammatory bowel disease. Here, a vicious cycle has been perpetuated. Because the intestine has been thoroughly emptied, a bowel movement is not possible for days. However, bulimarexics, assuming that they are constipated, resort to more laxatives. Such prolonged irritation and stimulation of the intestine can cause the muscles to become dependent upon laxatives for adequate contractile force. Thus, the laxative abuser will often feel bloated or experience gas or stomach pain. X rays often reveal a transient narrowing of the intestine similar to that of patients suffering from ulcerative colitis. Although in some cases these abnormalities have been partially reversed when the irritant laxatives were discontinued, this may not be possible in many cases, according to Drs. Jack R. Dreyfuss and Murray L. Janower, the editors of a 1980 book, *Radiology of the Colon.*

How can such serious problems develop? Quite simply, purging can become *habitual,* regardless of how it is accomplished. The purger is typically dehydrated and hungry. She is therefore likely to eat and drink more. after having done so she will usually feel full and then, of course, reinitiate the cycle by purging once again. In the process, the binge and the purge become associated with a multitude of environmental cues that soon come to elicit the urge to binge or purge.

Secondary Ammenorrhea

Secondary ammenorrhea or cessation of menstruation after having begun to menstruate is not unusual among bulimarexics. In many instances this is attributed to undernourishment. Dr. Rose Frisch has shown that established menstrual function is curtailed in women when fat levels drop below approximately 22 percent of body weight. Thus, fluctuation in body weight around this critical range may well account for the menstrual irregularity so often reported by bulimarexics, particularly those who rely heavily upon fasting and / or extreme dieting as means of purging. In addition, the menstrual cycle can be interrupted by environmental stress, which is, of course, a primary factor in bulimarexia. Thus, many bulimarexics report that menstrual bleeding is less associated with dramatic weight fluctations than it is with the stresses of daily living and the undernourishment precipitated by frequent purging. Regardless of the underlying cause, however, it is a well established fact that a causal relationship exists between body weight, stress, and the onset and regularity of menstruation. As Dr. Vincent points out in relation to dancers who binge and purge, " 'thinness'—in and of itself or along with the 'stresses' of dancing—may be responsible both for the delay in the onset of menstruation and for the lack of maintenance of a regular menstrual cycle."

Because bulimarexics who suffer from ammenorrhea and menstrual irregularities have avoided physicians and their symptoms have gone unrecognized, little longitudinal research has been devoted to the consequences of this phenomenon. What are the long-term effects on the reproductive system? Are fertility or childbearing affected? Does menstruation return spontaneously when proper nutrition and therapy are instituted? Definitive answers to these questions are not currently available and must rest on honest communication between bulimarexics and their doctors. We do know that many bulimarexics have begun to menstruate normally once they have abandoned their bizarre eating habits and purgative practices, while also learning alternative means of stress reduction. We are therefore optimistic and hope that women will begin to value themselves enough to talk freely with their physicians.

The following letter from one of our clients illustrates many of the problems and potential ramifications of binge-ing and purging. This woman agreed to let us use her history, as told in her own words:

"Dear Drs. White,

"For the first five of my seven years as a bulimarexic, I experienced fairly minor health problems. I had occasional dizzy spells, headaches, stomach cramps, and the obvious negative reactions from laxative abuse. However, the summer of my fifth year marked the beginning of serious problems that would increase until I finally gave up this abusive habit.

"I had been terribly depressed. I was in what I considered to be a 'fat' period. Liquid protein diets were the 'in' thing that summer and I felt this was my answer. I began ingesting supplements of this vile substance, but continued to use a diuretic as I felt this all-liquid diet would make me bloated. Needless to say, I was playing roulette! It was only a matter of time before I was so weak and lethargic I could barely function, even on a schedule of light activity. I became more depressed even though the sight of weight coming off usually boosted my spirits enough to keep up my abusive ritual.

"One day I was driving to visit my sister. I became so dizzy that my vision was blurred, and I began shaking. I actually feared for my life! I somehow managed to get to my sister's house, although the last thing I should have been doing was operating a car. I remember telling my sister I really needed a glass of orange juice. She asked me if I was sick. I looked terrible! All I could see was that I looked thin!! Anyway, I stayed at her house until I began feeling better and felt able to return home. As soon as I got home, however, I felt so faint that I was scared to be alone. I drove myself to the emergency room of the hospital. I told them I was having dizzy spells, felt faint, and just wanted to be sure I didn't have 'some sort of virus.' I was so good at concealing the cause of my suffering.

"The doctor on duty took my blood pressure, some blood samples, and made the routine checks that I guess all emergency patients receive. After a few minutes, the lab reports were back. The doctor looked at me and said, 'No wonder you feel so lousy, you're barely alive.' I knew he wasn't kidding. He then began to tell me that I had a potassium deficiency. I was anemic and lacking in all sorts of important minerals. I was so afraid of being 'discovered' that I took the news as if I had caught something dreadful from the air! He then began to ask me about my medical history—what had I possibly done to cause this reaction? I was a master at avoiding any answer which would implicate me as a laxative abuser. Finally, he asked the key question. 'Have you been dieting strenuously?' I was sure he knew enough from my lab reports to figure this one out. I decided to be partially honest. 'Well yes,' I answered, 'I have been dieting very seriously.' He then threw up his hands and in disgust said, 'You damn women and your diets, don't you know that your body must have a minimum of nutrients to survive?' I said yes, and that I should have been taking a vitamin supplement. He laughed and said that I'd have to take a lot more than a vitamin pill to regain normal status and proceeded to write my prescriptions for potassium supplements, megavitamins, iron, and folic acid.

"I left feeling relieved that I was still well enough to go home and not be hospitalized, but really shaken by the entire experience. I look back on that now and remember how relieved I was that he hadn't discovered that I was severely bulimarexic at that time. I was very careful after that. I took my medicine faithfully, went back for my check-up lab tests, and breathed a sign of relief. I did not, however, stop binge-ing and purging at that point. I just began to eat again, threw out the liquid protein, and purged less often for a while.

"Two years later, I began having difficulty when I urinated. Thinking I had a bladder infection or cystitis, I went to my doctor to have it checked out. When he looked at me, he said he didn't think I had a bladder infection but that I seemed to have a great deal of acidity in my urine, which caused the burning sensation I had been experiencing. He was also concerned that it might have something to do with a low grade infection which could have caused the urinary problem.

"I left his office in complete disgust. I had done this! I knew it was from abusing diuretics and laxatives. This was my breaking point. I had gone as far down as I could go. I was so depressed and disgusted with the entire habit that I was determined to turn my life and what health I had left around. I knew I had to get treatment.

"I stopped binge-ing on September 21, 1979, right after our workshop. I remember the date as one remembers something wonderful and looks toward each anniversary with anticipation. However, I had no way of knowing that my seven years of abuse would continue to plague me for sometime.

"Fifteen months after I had completely stopped binge-ing and purging, I had major abdominal surgery for a tumor. My immediate fear was that I had caused this with laxatives. I decided to tell all—to share my entire bulimarexic history with my physician. He was a wonderful listener. Patiently he sat as I went through my story. By the end I was crying. I remember telling him that for fifteen months I had been so 'good' and that I had to know if I had done this to myself. He told me that it was something that could never really be answered, but that the body has strange ways of scarring and healing itself after trauma. He said that although he wasn't sure if bulimarexia actually caused the tumor, he felt that through years of abuse of this area, I might have weakened it enough to make it more susceptible to injury or disease. He tried hard to reassure me that I had not necessarily done this to myself, but I am not convinced. Although my tumor was benign and I am now fully recovered, I can only hope that repercussions associated with bulimarexia are over. I write this in order that you might use it to help others before it is too late."

Unless the bulimarexic can be completely honest about the severity of her binge / purge behavior, she can anticipate little help. Many women have reached out to excellent physicians, psychologists, and nutritionists, but it is not enough for them merely to inform their doctors that they rely on laxatives, diuretics, or vomiting. Women report, "My doctor will not take me seriously." Inherent in this veiled plea for help is the hope that the doctor will somehow condone the aberrant behavior, and, in fact, that is often what happens. Take Eunice, for example. At a nationally recognized clinic, she was examined by no less than four specialists. Almost all of the adverse medical findings cited in this chapter were present, yet none of these top-flight specialists uncovered her eight-year history of binge-vomiting! Eunice was not dishonest—she "mentioned" vomiting to three of the four doctors, but she did not *emphasize* it. Instead of admitting to vomiting approximately two to three times daily after consuming an average of eight to ten thousand calories, Eunice merely stated that she *sometimes* felt bloated after overeating and would vomit uncontrollably. Physicians are not yet sophisticated about bulimarexia, despite the burgeoning interest resulting from articles in the lay press. They are skeptical—prone to shake their heads in disbelief. Psychological problems and the study of nutrition have only recently become a significant part of the medical school curriculum in the United States. Many doctors have learned to probe, yet they are also aware of the importance of establishing rapport in a relatively short period of time. This is not to excuse the physician who matter-of-factly dismisses important diagnostic cues with such statements as, "The way you look, you don't have to worry about your weight!" But doctors are not clairvoyant, nor can they be expected to be.

As a result of our group work, we have established a referral system with physicians and nurse-practitioners at Cornell. That system has now been extended to include others throughout the States. Some of those involved are practitioners; others are research clinicians; many were or are bulimarexic. All are interested in this pervasive problem and its medical ramifications. Soon medical journals will be publishing empirical studies about bulimarexia. At the moment, however, responsibility must rest with the bulimarexic and those to whom she turns in desperation. We would urge such potential sources of support to *insist* upon regular medical monitoring and to insure, whenever possible, that doctors, nutritionists, and therapists, are aware of the frequency and duration of binge-purge behavior. On the other hand, professionals who encounter these women must be more assertive, particularly during the initial interview, if treatment is to be effective. The first step must therefore involve early detection and referral to appropriate treatment resources.

CHAPTER 7

The Treatment of Bulimarexia

To laugh is to risk appearing the fool,
To weep is to risk appearing sentimental,
To reach out for another is to risk involvement,
To expose feelings is to risk exposing the self,
To place ideas and dreams before the crowd is to risk loss,
To love is to risk rejection,
To live is to risk dying,
To hope is to risk despair,
To try at all is to risk failure,
But risk we must,
Because the greatest hazard of all is to risk nothing,
For those who risk nothing, do nothing, have nothing, are nothing.

GROUP MEMBER

We have worked with over two thousand women struggling with bulimarexia, and we believe that bulimarexia is a learned behavior. It can therefore be unlearned. By behavior, we mean not only actions, but thought processes and attitudes as well. As with many behavioral problems, early detection often facilitates recovery in therapy. Those who came to us when they were just beginning to binge

and purge—and were frightened that they might continue—often were able to change their destructive eating
habits with relative ease. Some, though not all, could have
handled their problems themselves or with a minimum of
therapy if they had been familiar with the principles of our
treatment program. We hope that this chapter will prove
helpful to such women—and to the parents, husbands,
lovers, and friends who are wondering what they can do.

Many of the women we see have already had years of
individual psychotherapy. Often their therapists have
focused on deep-seated underlying causes, which did not
help the women with the here and now. Some were labeled
anorexic and were confronted with clinical descriptions that
were foreign and frightening. Others have continued to
feel bizarre and alone, even though they were told that
their behavior was not uncommon. And there are some
who had never admitted to their secret eating behavior. In
other words, they did not "own" their binge-ing and purging.

The bulimarexics we have met have attempted to deal
with their problems in a variety of treatment settings. Individual work with a male or a female therapist is the most
usual. Here a combination of behavioral, rational-emotive,
gestalt, interpersonal problem-solving, and assertiveness
training techniques seems most beneficial, especially when
the therapist understands the way most women are reared
in our culture. In one-to-one therapy, female therapists
may have better results, because women tend to relate to
and identify with one another, and also because bulimarexics have an overwhelming tendency to surrender their
power to men. In general, these are especially attractive
women who are "good patients" in the traditional sense.
They want to please, and they rarely challenge a male

therapist. As pointed out earlier, few bulimarexic women are completely honest about the frequency, intensity, and duration of the behaviors they yearn to alter.

As we reviewed the progress of these women, we came to feel that individual therapy was not the most effective treatment (in fact, it began to seem the least effective). Our exploratory work soon proved so revealing that we began more intensive group therapy as an alternative to individual work. Initially, our groups consisted of twelve to fifteen bulimarexics. We found that this number was too large and began limiting the group to no more than ten women. The group work is intensely demanding, requiring much "after hours" processing with regard to each participant. The group soon becomes cohesive so that short-term, intensive therapy is ideally suited to addressing specific goals. Since the women come from various areas of the country, there are also logistical and financial considerations, which include travel and leaving families and work responsibilities. In recent years, we have adopted a workshop format involving fifteen to twenty hours of therapy over a three-day period. This allows ample time for formal group work, informal risk taking outside of the group, and at the same time reinforces our belief that bulimarexia is a habit rather than a chronic disease process. Special attention is, of course, given to clarifying treatments goals and assuring that those who need follow-up and more extensive professional intervention can receive it.

Who should be treated in this type of group? We feel that the group should be composed of women who are truly bulimarexic. Women suffering from classic anorexia nervosa or obesity are not appropriate to this group experience. Their dynamics are quite different. They cannot identify with the bulimarexic and therefore run the risk of further alienation. Many are in need of medical management and, as such, should not be included.

It might be supposed that successful outcome in treatment is directly related to how long the destructive eating pattern has been going on, to the intensity of gorging and purging, and to the methods these women use to purge. While it is generally true that women in the early stages of bulimarexia recover more quickly, two factors seem far more relevant. The first involves the *level of commitment to change* the woman possesses when she enters treatment. Second, but of equal importance, are the *strategies* she employs to overcome bulimarexia. What can she do in the face of anxiety? What can she substitute for binge eating? If the woman can call upon more productive strategies to cope with the stresses of daily life, she is on her way to recovery. The commitment to initiate and maintain personal growth through alternative behaviors is therefore crucial.

Naming this behavior *bulimarexia* was not something we wanted to do because such labeling could, in and of itself, be harmful. Labels, unless clearly defined in terms of precise behaviors, often serve as a refuge. They symbolize safe edifices behind which a person can hide and wait to be "cured." In order to avoid this, let us review the primary characteristics of bulimarexia, so that women who are suffering from classic anorexia and obesity do not seek treatment that was not intentionally designed for them.

First, the bulimarexic alternately binges on food and then purges, typically by self-induced vomiting, or by abuse of laxatives or diuretics. Although fasting can be another method of purging, it is far less prevalent and should not be confused with the typical anorexic pattern in which the *major emphasis is on starvation*. Second, the bulimarexic is obsessed with not getting fat. For her, actual body weight is far less important than her body proportions and how *she sees herself*. Self-esteem is based primarily upon how she feels she looks, so that the successes (or failures) of her life are measured by this yardstick.

MYTHS ABOUT BULIMAREXIA

When we began our group work, we soon found that most women were eager to share their histories. It was as if they were trying to shock each other, to outdo one painful story with another. At the same time, it was clear that they had certain misconceptions about their binge / purge behavior. The following are the most usual—and the most crucial:

1. *Bulimarexia is a disease, a mental illness.* To categorize this syndrome as a disease is dangerous. Many women who engage in this behavior would like to believe that a disease or illness has overtaken them. We are convinced that bulimarexia is a learned behavior—a *habit* that can prove exceedingly difficult to give up. However, if it is learned it can be unlearned, utilizing basic principles and techniques to be discussed in this chapter. Those who insist that the binge / purge syndrome is a disease run the risk of believing that someone does "it" to them and someone must cure them. In any case, the "victim" is off the hook!

2. *It has taken years for me to become bulimarexic; therefore, it will take years to stop.* This self-defeating philosophy only results in a stronger commitment to a bulimarexic lifestyle. By clinging to such an attitude, the woman allows herself no chance to try other, possibly more productive behaviors. With help, most women can acknowledge the irration-

ality of this "years-to-stop" premise and develop more realistic alternatives to stress than binge-ing. We often point out that women who have been chronic bingers for fifteen to twenty years have curtailed or eliminated the behavior in a few months. Women who have been successful are usually eager to share their experiences with others still engaged in the struggle. We use their valuable suggestions in our group by way of letters, tapes, and, whenever possible, direct involvement. In this way we can *show* rather than tell the struggling bulimarexic that her basic belief system is not only in error, but is serving to hold her back.

3. *Unless I understand why I binge and purge, I'll never be able to give it up.* Although the pursuit of underlying causes is fascinating and occasionally rewarding, it has typically resulted in extreme frustration and failure for the vast majority of bulimarexics. In fact, their obsession with *why* they binge and purge consumes most of their valuable energy, leaving them especially vulnerable to continued failure. As an alternative, we invite them to abandon this elusive pursuit and join us in concentrating on *what they get* from gorging and purging. What are the pay-offs? How is the behavior serving them? Is it really *helping* them to avoid pain, responsibility, and / or intimacy? Does the binge and purge actually serve to punish others or are they really defeating themselves over and over again? Since behavior is purposive, we emphasize that a person does not typically adhere to a particular behavior unless something is derived from it. Shifting the emphasis from *why* the woman is binge-ing and purging to *what* reward the behavior is offering allows her to discover, often for the first time, *how* bulimarexia is serving her.

4. *If I'm to give up gorging and purging, I must do so on my own.* Such a belief, admirable as it may seem at first glance,

has inhibited growth and development for countless buli-marexic women. Although self-reliance is in line with con-temporary feminist psychology, it is inappropriate in this particular context. The bulimarexic woman, in the throes of her difficulties, quite simply is not capable of sustaining herself independently. She is, in fact, *most vulnerable* when she is alone! Thus, it makes little sense to ask her to rely exclusively upon her own resources. Since the bulimarexic rarely binges or purges in the presence of others, we stren-uously encourage her to develop sources of support, often with other group members, and to set up goals (goal con-tracts) with these individuals. These contracts must be spe-cific and easily evaluated on a regular basis. The people selected for support, the nature of the contract, and the way progress is assessed are crucial. For example, it is not enough for the woman simply to ask a friend to "be there when I need you." This is far too ambiguous a contract. Instead, when the bulimarexic feels that the person she has in mind is willing to offer support and capable of doing so, she must then check this out with that person. If the chosen friend is another bulimarexic, the contract must be initiated with care. Because of their pervasive people-pleasing tendency, most bulimarexics will try to help even when they feel overwhelmed and incapable. Thus, it would be wise to assess the situation realistically before making an explicit contractual agreement. Furthermore, contract-ing with only *one* person is unwise. That person may not be available for support at that particular time, which may lead to an irresistible urge to binge. This can often be avoided by acknowledging the potential problem and developing flexible contracts with a few friends as back-ups.

It is important for the bulimarexic woman to be exact in

informing her potential sources of support about her *specific needs*. Take the example of Karla, who had been living by herself for almost a year and who had a history of extreme binge-ing alone in her apartment, often for days. When she left the group, Karla had decided to call either Jenny, Laura, or Alice *only* when she had exhausted all of her own strategies to ward off binge-ing. Weeks after her experience in the group, Karla was faced with a number of anxiety-arousing situations. After several unsuccessful attempts at coping, she felt depleted and in need of support. Her first call went unanswered; Jenny was out. In the past, this would have led to a binge; however, because Karla had agreed to reach out to others, she immediately called Laura. This time she connected. But Laura was having an argument with her husband and, since their original contract was predicated on honest communication, she informed Karla that she could not deal with additional pressure at that point. Laura asked Karla to call back the next morning.

Karla was frantic, yet she understood. Before calling Alice, she decided to write down her feelings, to clarify what she needed at this crucial time. The bottom line was reassurance about a painful decision she had recently made to abandon a relationship with a man that seemed to be going nowhere. The sense of isolation, aloneness, and inadequacy that she was feeling terrified her. She needed to feel connected to someone—or something. Reminding herself that she was under considerable stress, Karla made an appointment at a local health spa instead of raiding the refrigerator. Afterwards, she telephoned Jenny, who had returned home. They met later, and Jenny, listening intently, genuinely reassured Karla that she was right to end the relationship. Jenny also pointed out that such a decision was not irreversible and could be reevaluated at a later date. Most important, Jenny marveled at Karla's strength and ingenuity in avoiding gorging under pressure. Thus, both women maintained an honest, supportive stance. Karla showed herself and her friend that she could avoid binge-ing and could reach out for specific help even in extreme anxiety. In retrospect, Karla realized that despite her attempts to cope, she had panicked prematurely, reaching out before doing her "homework" and clarifying in writing what she felt she needed.

The next day Laura called Karla, having worked through her crisis with her husband. When Laura heard of Karla's success, she was equally genuine in reinforcing her friend. There was no need for Laura to apologize for the previous evening, since openness had been a condition of their contract.

It is unfair and potentially self-defeating for bulimarexics to ask for help and then expect others to know precisely how to respond. Relatives and close friends often feel that they were at least partially responsible for the initiation and / or maintenance of the woman's behavior, and their guilt and helplessness can make them reluctant to support her when she makes strides toward recovery. However, those closest to the bulimarexic need to feel that they are part of her success experiences and the ensuing recovery process. Unless they do, sabotage is likely, even though not intended. This sabotage can be subtle, as in the case of Claire, who moved out of her parent's home and returned to report good progress only to find both parents unwilling to trust that the gains would be permanent. In other instances, damage can be more overt. Janie's husband insisted that she eat alone each evening in order to demonstrate that she was completely cured. During this time, Janie said that her husband was quite punitive and demanding, as if he were "invested in keeping me a prisoner to bulimarexia." Obviously, the husband's attitude was not helpful, but Janie had not indicated exactly what she expected of him.

5. *As a bulimarexic I am powerless in the face of food.* This assumption feeds directly into the bulimarexic's sense of learned helplessness. It is not only illogical, but it successfully prevents the woman from self-motivation. Fortunately, this is the easiest assumption to dispel. Former patients who have been chronic bingers and purgers and who have, within a few weeks or months, developed the capacity to enjoy a palatable meal prove that it can be done.

The sense of powerlessness so familiar to anorexics and bulimarexics is often reinforced by popular articles about eating disorders. An article in the *New York Times* a few years ago referred to anorexics as "victims of the disease." Another, in *People* magazine in late 1981, carried the headline: "A Dangerous Eat-&-Purge Disorder Called Bulimia Strikes Young Women." Even more devastating was a 1981 article in *Time* magazine that indicated that "there were no known cures" for bulimia. Thus, the language used to describe these syndromes can inadvertently heighten a despair that is already extreme.

6. *When I stop binge-ing and purging, everything will be fine.* This naïve view either results in consistent disappointment and more frequent binge-ing, or it lets the woman "off the hook." There is no way that this expectation can be fulfilled. Furthermore, such a belief holds the *syndrome* accountable rather than the *person* who chooses to engage in binge / purge behavior. It is a not so subtle trick that the bulimarexic plays on herself and others. By maintaining that bulimarexia—that insidious, uncontrollable disease

process—makes her life miserable—the woman makes a commitment to despair. To believe that life will be trouble-free when she stops binge-ing is an excellent way of insuring that binge-ing will continue with a vengeance. After all, who among us is capable of controlling life so as to avoid discomfort completely? It is not coincidental that the bulimarexic often adheres to this myth, however, As mentioned earlier, she is a perfectionist interested in avoiding pain. And she will not allow herself even one mistake! She may be able to avoid binge-ing for weeks or months, but *one mistake* usually results in a return to extreme binge / purge behavior.

She is really saying, "Unless I am guaranteed that my life will be trouble-free when I stop binge-ing and purging, I will not give it up." Many a bulimarexic has admitted to this with a twinkle in her eye! This is a good beginning, for unless she is capable of "owning" the behavior, there is little she can do about it.

INDIVIDUAL THERAPY
WITHIN A GROUP CONTEXT

Although bulimarexic women are willing to identify with one another, they soon become aware that they are dissimilar in many ways. If such differences are not acknowledged, group disharmony can ensue. Group members may indicate that they do not feel "like everyone else here," claiming that their binges are not as severe, that their lifestyles are quite different, and that differences in age serve to separate them from other members. They are, of course, correct when they point out these differences. However, such observations in no way negate the therapy process.

What is crucial, then, is to *individualize* the treatment program for each group participant. Unless each woman is allowed to feel her individuality as an asset, she may well resist help through therapy yet remain in the group. Her presence then becomes a deterrent to the process of change. If we can redirect attention toward comon goals, considerable vicarious learning can take place.

Focusing on the "pay-offs" derived from bulimarexia often serves to unite the group. For there are very few pay-offs. In brief, gorging and purging come to be seen as either avoidance behaviors or as means of punishment. For some, it is the avoidance of intimacy, for others, the avoidance of success. Still others use binge-ing and purging as a way of avoiding failure. Another contingent of bulimarexic woman, particularly those in their late teens and early twenties, use binge-ing and purging to elicit attention and punish parents and others. In many such cases, the family is well aware of the bulimarexia and may even watch helplessly while the woman binges. A young woman may binge in order to avoid the awesome pursuit of success and, at the same time, cause her parents, who have consistently urged her to do well in all she encounters, to feel guilty. Another woman, on the verge of success in school or in the work world, may return to severe binge-ing out of fear of failure and, at the same time, punish her husband who, she feels, has not supported her in some important way.

When several group members have identified what maintains their binge-ing, they usually begin to identify with one another. Their sense of sisterhood and comaraderie is thus enhanced. It is not absolutely necessary for each woman to discover what she is deriving from her destructive behavior. Some are not ready to acknowledge this, some feel incapable of doing so, and others already know, but have done nothing to effect change. Those who do know, often begin to consider alternatives to binge-ing. Those who do not can observe those who do. Later, they too may be able to address this particular issue. It is especially important not to convey the notion that insight into the pay-off is necessary before the basic binge / purge cycle can be altered. At least 25 percent of the women we have worked with never identified their pay-offs within the group yet later were able to curtail or eliminate their binge / purge pattern on their own. Interviews with one hundred such women suggest that most of-them (usually after the group experience) made major modifications in the way they adapted to life situations only to realize that the new behavior served them far better than binge-ing. As might be expected, these women were generally less animated and verbal during our formal group therapy sessions.

REWRITING THE SCRIPT

Certain negative concepts make up the life script of the bulimarexic. A new understanding of the concept of *irreversibility* often helps to move women beyond their eating impasse. We emphasize that there are few behaviors that are irreversible and invite the women to explore new ways of dealing with their anxiety. We point out that their old ways do not appear to be working, so why not give some new ones a try? Unless the new ways are more palatable and productive, they always have the option of returning to binge-ing. What we are asking for is a commitment to a new strategy. We caution the women that anything new will feel unfamiliar. The new and unfamiliar can be uncomfortable for any of us and particularly so for the bulimarexic.

Most bulimarexics will wholeheartedly agree that their old ways have not been helpful and are therefore willing to explore new means of coping with the stress and anxiety that characteristically lead to a binge. Such a commitment thereby forces them to confront two major deterrents to psychological growth that not only characterize the bulimarexic, but are frequently present in all of us.

In dealing with the stresses and anxieties that lead to binge-ing, the bulimarexic has *learned to avoid pain at all costs*. If she is to change, she must learn to use painful thoughts as *motivators* rather than as excuses to binge. Pain is a precursor of change, particularly for those who are committed to gaining strength. Even a brief sojourn into our past will remind us that those experiences of which we are most proud can typically be traced to painful throughts and acts that we used to motivate risk taking. We therefore emphasize the importance of reevaluating each woman's methods of coping with pain by helping her to identify and troubleshoot her avoidance patterns. For example, Shelley, a "former" athlete, had decided that instead of competing and risking the pain of losing, she would simply avoid competitive sports. Before long, she felt that she rarely enjoyed any activities with other people and claimed that she was bored and becoming more reclusive.

Shelley was persuaded to join a bowling team, a sport she had previously enjoyed until the team members urged her to compete for team captain. In retrospect, she admitted that even if she had been able to control her anxiety and deal with her rivals' bantering, she did not want to be captain. She was not ready for the limelight, despite her obvious skill as a bowler. Now, when she was asked to "rehearse for catastrophe," Shelley said that her greatest fear was that she would be judged adversely, especially by "expert bowlers." Actually, she was her own worst critic, constantly alluding to her imagined ineptitudes. Other group members soon helped her to see how she set herself up for ridicule—how she planted these thoughts in others. Shelley agreed to try to substitute more realistic messages to herself when she was bowling. Such statements as, "I know I'm going to blow it now," "This is an impossible spare," and "I'm sure Sarah will never forgive me if we don't win" were rephrased as "I'll give it my best now," "I'll try and pick up this spare by . . . ," and "Sarah seems so intent upon winning—I feel that pressure and am therefore going to *ask her* what she's feeling."

By ceasing to anticipate the worst, Shelley was able to enjoy healthy competition once more while satisfying her need to be gregarious, which had gone unfilled for nearly five years.

Most bulimarexics also live either in the past or in the future. When confronted by a situation that is moderately challenging, they look to the past for coping strategies (binge-ing) or look ahead and rehearse for tragedy (nothing will work out). Since the past cannot be changed and the future is, for the most part, unpredictable (or contingent upon what one does in the moment), we encourage group members to replace these habits with a *present, action-oriented* attitude. The women learn to talk to themselves *in the moment* and to engage their "old" part and their "new" part in a dialogue at the moment pain begins. Such "top-dog / underdog" techniques forces an important dialogue that is first undertaken aloud in the group so that all can help the woman to deal with unsure and irrational beliefs that have reinforced topdog for so long.

By the way of illustration, consider Diane, a "5 o'clock binger." Each afternoon after work, Diane headed straight for the supermarket. When she claimed that she was "magnetized by the place," we encouraged the pessimistic part of her (topdog) to indulge in this belief. Underdog was then invited to speak. The quality and intensity of this monologue was, at first, pathetic. Group members joined to bolster underdog and with time and support, Diane began to invest this neglected yet vital part of herself with more energy. She soon recognized that topdog statements were based almost exclusively upon *past* and *future* considerations, whereas underdog was present-oriented. Topdog statements were loaded with "can'ts" and similar pessimistic beliefs based upon past failures, or they reflected expectations that were essentially unwarranted (*"Yes,* I could try that, *but* I doubt it will work"). Underdog statements ("I want to try an alternate route home") reflected new strategies that could be undertaken in the present. As such, they could be evaluated and, if necessary, troubleshot. Diane saw the irrationality of topdog and, with the help of the group, began to confront this element before succumbing to its toxic message. By the end of the group experience, Diane was reexamining her script and rewriting it. Underdog was gaining strength and was consistently reinforced by all of us. Thus, unless the bulimarexic is willing to ask "What tense am I in?" (present, rather than past or future) when confronted by anxiety-arousing stimuli, she will, more often than not, follow her old script and fail to grow.

Another stumbling block to change involves what we call the "bionic woman syndrome." Bulimarexics expect perfection. They may, for instance, remain binge-free for weeks, only to encounter problems that trigger overeating.

After one lapse, rather than scrutinizing the setback and learning from it, they classically revert to full-fledged gorging and purging. What is important here is their unwillingness or inability to reward themselves for their obvious strength over a period of weeks and to profit from that single mistake by troubleshooting what led to overeating. Through "homework assignments" that involve specific scenarios that set the stage for a binge, the bulimarexic brings to the group a number of alternatives that can then be examined. Each woman thus rewrites her script in a trial and error fashion. Because *she* is the principal author, she often overcomes resistance to change and has more energy to devote to this valuable and rewarding pursuit. In Shelley's situation, homework logically followed from the role plays centering around bowling. In fact, upon leaving the group one evening, she and three group members engaged in a shuffleboard contest. All eyes were upon her, especially when game pressure was high. Although Shelley did poorly and lost a game for her team, she performed well in other ways. By self-monitoring her pessimistic statements and avoiding interpretation and analysis of the other women, she not only delighted in the excitement of the game, but began to see how she could develop intimacy by sharing her feelings with her partner.

GOAL CONTRACTING

Each group member establishes her own goals, which she articulates in a specific fashion. She is now making an overt commitment in the presence of others with whom she has begun to feel comfortable. It is important at this point to clarify the difference between a *goal* and an *expec-*

tation. Quite simply, an expectation implies an outcome. A goal does not; it merely represents a commitment to *try.* Since most bulimarexic women have defeated themselves countless times as a result of unrealistic expectations, we ask them to reassess this self-sabotage maneuver. Each woman reviews the most effective process she has employed to give up binge-ing and purging. Invariably, someone will describe a time when she was binge-free for weeks only to encounter real difficulties that precipitated a relapse. Upon discovering that their expectation was that they would *never* binge again, the women soon realize that such perfection-ism assures failure in the long run. Statements like "I'll *never* binge again" or 'I'm giving this up *forever*" can only hamper well-intentioned bulimarexics.

This is also true of negative expectations. For example, "I know as hard as I try I'll never be completely binge-free" is a commitment to failure. Not surprisingly, buli-marexic women often say: "I must gain total self-control"; "I will no longer feel anxious and vulnerable with men"; "I should establish friendships with women without ever being competitive and mistrustful"; and "I must under-stand why I binge and purge." How much better if these expectations become goals that can be restated as: "I want to learn *what* I am getting from allowing myself to binge and purge"; "I want to try to communicate in an honest, straightforward fashion, especially with men to whom I am attracted"; "I want to take more risks with friendship, especially with women whom I admire"; and "I want to focus on *how* binge-ing and purging are serving me in a variety of contexts." Now they are beginning to think in terms of how, when, and where they might accomplish specific objectives.

There should be a *number* of alternatives rather than a

single alternative to binge-ing, since no one behavior is powerful enough to displace binge-ing under stress. Again, the group process is helpful because of the similarity between one woman's particular avoidance pattern and those of other women. Through this problem-solving approach, the woman who is less likely to verbalize can feel a part of the group process. Even so, each woman must ultimately try some alternative ways of coping. Outside the group, all group members are aware of the other participants' specific contracts to take risks with new behavior. As therapists, we summarize individual goals and encourage the women to act as facilitators for each other. The time the women spend together doing "homework" in the evenings and throughout the day is therefore as therapeutic as the time spent in formal session. As did Shelley, many women actively explore a number of alternatives and experience the consequences directly. Those who participate in these exercises often stimulate other, less motivated women toward their goals.

Tina, one of the onlookers in the shuffleboard incident, wrote recently regarding her progress. Although she never admitted it during our group work, she had always felt guilty about being athletic, especially when she competed with men to whom she was attracted. Feeling that all men would reject her if she won, she would often hold back in order that they might excel. Shelley's new strategy had impressed Tina. She respected Shelley, and they became friends. Upon returning home, after some deliberation, Tina called a man who she liked and admired. They went skiing, and she really "went for it." Much to her delight, he was impressed. With time, they became ski partners, friends, and, ultimately, lovers. Tina kept in touch with Shelley, whom she occasionally used as a "sounding board for my new strategies." Although her relationship with this man eventually came to an end, Tina continued to perform to the best of her abilities. She recognized that certain men might be alienated by her competence, but, more important, she discovered that others found her irresistible! Tina is now married and attending medical school. As she pointed out, "It only took eleven months to beat bulimarexia after I began to be real rather than ideal." Showing the bulimarexic that what she *does* determines her identity and ultimately her sense of self is far more effective than simply telling her. We therefore place great emphasis upon helping women to discover that *they are what they do,* not what they think and feel.

Bulimarexic women *do not know how to say no.* By saying "yes" when they really mean "no," they accumulate sufficient justifications for a later binge. This binge is "OK" because they have paid their dues by being available and accommodating when, in fact, they were really overloaded. The binge thus serves as a reward for being dishonest and accepting responsibility that they know they do not wish to handle. In their view, an honest, straightforward statement such as "I'm unable to help right now," is simply not polite. It is not feminine! In short, to say "no" when you do not wish to engage in a particular activity is less desirable than possibly offending others and assuring a binge.

In this same vein, the majority of bulimarexics have trouble accepting a compliment. This is easily illustrated in the group, particularly when we, as therapists, offer positive feedback. Although this behavior is understandable in light of the bulimarexic's poor self-concept, the inability or unwillingness to be rewarded stunts psychological growth. The occasional, dishonest transactions that these women allow themselves only set the stage for binge-ing. Elaine was classic in this regard. Beautiful, talented, and successful, she was a master of the "Yes, but . . ." game. Offer her a genuine compliment and she would say, "Yes, but look at how weak and pathetic I am." At first, group members were sympathetic and continued to point out Elaine's assets, but they grew more and more frustrated as she continued to deprecate herself. This was perhaps best illustrated when we invited Elaine to troubleshoot (identify self-sabotaging statements) in the following roleplay between Bill and Marlene:

MARLENE: You don't like the way I'm dressed, do you?

BILL: Yes, I think you look great!

MARLENE: Come on, Bill, I know you think this skirt looks foolish.

BILL: It's not my favorite, but I think you look great tonight.

MARLENE: See, you're just trying to make me feel good!

BILL: I'm being honest with you, Marlene. You really look fine.

MARLENE: But not great—you can tell me; I know I don't look great, right?

BILL: Well, whatever you say, but I still feel that you look very nice and I'm hungry, so let's go to the dinner party.

MARLENE: Hold on, I want to change into something else. I can't stand going out when you don't like the way I'm dressed.

What is preventing Marlene from feeling good about herself? This was the question we asked. Now that she was outside the experience, Elaine could zero in on Marlene's self-defeating style. Others were also helpful, particularly during time outside the group, in pointing out Elaine's pervasive habit and refusing to reinforce it. After consistent exposure to honest feedback, Elaine altered her put-down messages to herself and began to acknowledge her good qualities. Several months later, she accepted a modeling contract in order to obtain enough money to attend college and begin a career as a physical therapist. Before the group experience, she had refused to "use my looks and figure instead of my mind." Now that she has explored a creative compromise, Elaine is no longer so myopic. She still binges occasionally, but has given up the major "racket" that led to regular binge / purge behavior, perpetuated a poor self-image, and gave her an opportunity to get off the hook.

REDEFINING FEMININITY

Once the toxic behaviors described above are exposed, group members directly confront the major precursors of binge / purge behavior. As women in our culture, they have unwittingly taken the posture of accommodation to its extreme. What follows is a redefinition of the feminine role.

At this point, Marlene works alone with the group. The issues addressed depend on the particular make-up of each group. When it is composed of younger women, struggles for independence and problems with parents are often crucial. Groups of older, married women and mothers present different topics for examination.

Because of their basically dishonest lifestyle, intimacy is rare among bulimarexics. Few have close female friends, and those who do feel intensely competitive and mistrustful of female companionship. One of the primary goals of this segment of treatment is to facilitate open communication. Encouraging women to like and respect others with similar problems often serves to enhance their self-esteem. This is particularly important for bulimarexic women since they tend to relinquish their power, particularly in the presence of men. To illustrate this point, Marlene will frequently draw from earlier interactions that took place when Bill was present. She demonstrates how group members almost invariably vied for the attention of the male therapist, even attributing change to *his* invention. Many are, in effect, acting as though they are in dire need of being rescued. However, women must develop their own strengths and capacity for growth if they are to achieve a sense of self. Oneness must precede twoness. And there are golden opportunities available to every woman, thanks to feminist principles and awareness. Thus, one goal of our treatment involves encouraging strong feelings of sisterhood among group participants. Reactions from scores of women over the years suggest that such a bond can be therapeutic in and of itself. This sense of connectedness ensures a support structure that sustains the women during the initial difficult months after treatment.

As part of our treatment program, group participants from the same geographical area are asked to room together. In addition, they are encouraged to spend time together outside of the group. Those who report increased feelings of self-worth because they are able to help and encourage one another begin to demonstrate less reliance upon us, the therapists.

Most bulimarexics have few women in their lives they can admire. Part of Marlene's function with the group involves sharing her personal struggles with the same issues of self-worth, body image, and acceptability to men. Group members are often curious to know whether Marlene was herself a bulimarexic. Some women seize on the fact that she was not. Some even claim she cannot understand their problem and are reluctant to acknowledge her insights. By describing her own imperfections, Marlene counteracts the concept of "bionic woman" and helps to dispel the myth of perfectionism. Group members can relate to her as a professional woman with her own problems. The myth of uniqueness is also exposed when it becomes apparent that all of the women have shared common feelings, mistakes, and failures. This kind of communication often gives the women a powerful sense of hope. They become aware that a different kind of future is possible.

Bulimarexics traditionally believe that a man's love will transform their lives by relieving them of responsibility. Each woman is therefore asked to assess what heterosexual relationships have meant to her. Many discover that by relinquishing responsibility for decision-making, they have not only undermined their self-concept, but have alienated the men with whom they were involved. Often, with the help of the group, these women are able to understand the anger, resentment, and disillusionment expressed by fathers, husbands, and boyfriends.

Louise is a prime example. In order to avoid criticism, she gradually turned over her responsibilities to other people, one by one. First, although she had a degree in mathematics, she stopped writing checks when her husband complained because of an occasional overdraft. Then she stopped helping her daughter with her homework, turning this responsibility over to her eighteen-year-old son. She even gave up her part-time job as an instructor of gymnastics after a youngster, known for her caustic tongue, made a disparaging remark to her. In the process of diminishing herself, Louise became physically inactive and resorted to binge-ing and purging in hopes of retaining her figure. Her husband, son, and daughter, frustrated in their attempts to intervene in what they considered "menopausal depression," became more and more resentful of and angry with Louise, finally insisting that she commit herself to a psychiatric hospital. After two months she was discharged and referred to us.

Upon entering the group, Louise was initially treated with compassion by the other women. But soon they began to realize that they had trapped themselves and, at the therapist's suggestion, initiated a role play based upon Louise's description of her former lifestyle at home. Anger and resentment emerged and Louise, for the first time, realized that her gradual isolation from the family had precipitated much of the unpleasantness. Louise realized that she had become bored and was particularly vulnerable to binge-ing. Nevertheless, she felt inept and unsure of her most basic skills. In order to assess this view of herself, Louise was asked to prepare a "mini-lecture" involving basic concepts in geometry. It so happened that Regina, a college sophomore and a group member, was having difficulty in a math course and had brought her textbook along. The following morning, after about an hour's preparation, Louise gave her lecture and was magnificent! Even the dullest among us was able to follow her succinct, professional presentation. More important, Louise was proud of herself. This proved to be a new beginning for a woman who, two months previously, had been hospitalized. Contracts involving more assertive behavior were then initiated and tested within and outside the group and later at home with her husband, who was described as domineering and critical yet eager to save their marriage. Louise has begun to "take back her power," but not without considerable struggle. At present, she is working on a master's degree, and she has been binge-free for over two years.

In addition to risk-taking and assuming responsibility, issues involving sexuality are often primary during the all-women part of the group. Many of the women admit to being nonorgasmic despite the fact that they crave sexual contact. They anticipate intercourse with trepidation, feeling inadequate and incapable of satisfying their partners (or themselves). Major emphasis is therefore placed upon how to communicate and thereby build a good sexual partnership. The first step in this venture is to examine the self-loathing these women feel toward their bodies.

For bulimarexics, the pursuit of slimness is their raison d' etre. A common fantasy is that their lives will change when they are *thin enough*. In dispelling this fantasy, showing beats telling once again. Women in the group who are slightly overweight quickly perceive that exceedingly slim and beautiful group members also feel worthless and unlovable. The women begin to see that *they*, not men, turn themselves into sexual objects through a narcissistic preoccupation with weight and appearance. As they share their perceptions of their bodies and hear comments about the distorted images, many veer toward a more realistic assessment of their physicalities.

Those who are slightly overweight no longer exaggerate their flaws, and those slightly underweight seem to accept the need to add weight in a gradual, healthy manner. Marlene encourages the women to engage in sports and other physical activities. Emphasis is thereby shifted from inactivity or compulsive attempts to rid the body of dreaded calories to deriving pleasure from one's body.

Much of this session involves goal contracting, some of

which includes important issues concerning men that can be undertaken with Bill at a later point. For example, during a group session, Gloria disclosed that she had been faking orgasm for fear of offending or losing her boyfriend. She also believed there was something wrong with her because she required sustained clitoral stimulation to become sexually aroused. Because she made no effort to communicate her fears to her boyfriend, he had assumed that everything was all right. Group members were able to assure Gloria that she was not abnormal.

At first, Gloria was embarrassed to discuss her sexual feelings so openly. However, as the other women spoke up, Gloria relaxed and expressed a desire to confront this issue in the group. A contract was therefore initiated, and Gloria was asked to participate in an "empty chair" exercise by imagining that her boyfriend was sitting in the chair. Gloria was then asked to try new ways of conversing about sex with him. This was exceedingly difficult for her. She stumbled and muddled, was incoherent at one point, and became frustrated again and again. Such "mistakes" were identified as typical by other group members, and Gloria eventually discovered what she wanted to say to her boyfriend. She found that she liked herself best when she got rid of "sweetsy pie" and was "straight and direct." She had discovered one of the great yet elusive pay-offs associated with being authentic and real.

Gloria continued to work on this issue with Bill when he rejoined the group. Since her boyfriend was exceedingly controlling, Bill's dialogue with Gloria was deliberately "macho" in order to assess her proposed strategies in the face of stress. Gloria fared quite well under this "rough handling," which helped her to realize that she was not as fragile as she had believed and therefore *acted*. Such scenarios underline the importance of the all-women part of the group. Few of these issues would have been raised had a male been present.

Assertiveness training is central to our treatment because bulimarexics are eager to appease others and to avoid conflict at any cost. Unfortunately, this kind of behavior is generally approved of and considered socially acceptable: the woman who is agreeable and ameliorating is a "good" friend, wife, or daughter. In the long run, however, appeasement results in loss of self-esteem and suppressed anger. Again, we have a classic precursor of binge-ing. It is our task as therapists to help women develop more appropriate coping skills. Parent-daughter issues, husband-wife transactions, and mother-child problems are therefore played out to develop more active and responsible alternatives to the old ways of handling conflicts. Each woman can then demonstrate and practice these new alternatives and learn to accept the validity of her own emotions. The following example illustrates the importance of assertiveness and helps to define what the term "assertion" really means.

Jennifer bitterly complained that she was unable to sustain relationships with men. What she wanted more than anything was an intimate relationship. Because she had never had intimacy with a man, she considered herself a failure. Over the years she found herself dissatisfied with men in one way or another and would typically end relationships in the initial stages. After listening carefully, group members noted that Jennifer had certain mistaken beliefs about the way women should act with men. For example, she obviously equated assertion with aggression and thought that nonassertion meant that she was being polite and considerate. In defending herself, Jennifer

spoke repeatedly about "not wanting to hurt his feelings."
Not surprisingly, Jennifer's encounters with men were dis-
tressingly repetitive. Because she was strikingly beautiful,
men were attracted to her. When a man tried to find out
if she was similarly attracted to him, she would typically
encourage him (even if she did not care for the man), not
wishing to "hurt him." Having received what he felt were
assurances, the man would pursue her more actively. Jennifer would then begin to "turn off" and, at the same time,
hate herself for her deception. However, she typically
placed the blame on the man for "pushing her" and developed even more devious maneuvers to avoid other men.
She invested an inordinate amount of time into such
demoralizing encounters so that, in the end, most of the
men felt deeply hurt and "taken." Jennifer felt increasingly guilty and concluded that she was incapable of intimacy with men.

Jennifer was asked to try to communicate her feelings in
a role play, with Bill acting the part of her current boyfriend. At first, Jennifer had great difficulty maintaining
eye contact with Bill. She hunched her shoulders, covered
her mouth with her hand, and displayed a variety of nervous, distracting gestures. Her speech pattern was hesitant, with many pauses, and she acted in a subservient, self-
effacing manner. Group members commented on Jennifer's mannerisms and described how she seemed to them.
Marlene then reenacted and exaggerated some of Jennifer's responses in an attempt to *show* her how she appeared
to others. Next some of the other group members mod-
eled several alternative ways of relating and gently prod-
ded Jennifer to take some risks and try some new ways of
responding on her own. This was difficult for her, but after
two or three attempts, she was more animated, alive, and

self-confident. She admitted that, despite its unfamiliarity, "it felt good to be honest." A few group members and Bill spontaneously expressed delight and respect for Jennifer's behavior, and she began to see the benefits of assertiveness. After all, she hated herself for being dishonest and constantly put herself down for her lack of courage. Jennifer's work, however, had just begun. Later that evening, she practiced her new communication skills with a young man she met at a pub. She stumbled and was unsure of what to say and how to say it, but in the process she learned that she was not as fragile as she had supposed. About a year later, Jennifer wrote of the fun and friendships she was having with men. They found her openness refreshing and rare. Bolstered by these successes, she became more and more committed to risk taking rather than to helplessness.

Like Jennifer, few women will need to binge if they have more productive ways of identifying and satisfying their needs. They will no longer find it necessary to stuff themselves to ward off anger if they can acknowledge and express it more appropriately. The same applies to all forms of stress. Instead of binge-ing as an escape from studying, a break in routine becomes possible. Instead of turning to food out of boredom and / or loneliness, women can acknowledge their loneliness and learn to socialize. Instead of binge-ing to escape from uncomfortable situations, they can discover how to say "no."

NEW STRATEGIES IN OLD SITUATIONS

The bulimarexic is typically most vulnerable to binge-ing and purging when she is *alone*. As pointed out earlier, it is important for these women to avoid being alone, at difficult times and places or with people who invariably elicit anxiety. Many women are likely to binge on the job. They keep junk foods concealed in their desks, cars, or other convenient places where the hoard is not readily detectable. They can cut down on or eliminate sneak binge-ing if they make a deliberate effort not to be alone. Also, it is not possible to binge "uncontrollably" if there is nothing to consume. Thus, at the very least, the binger who is truly committed to alternatives will reach out to others for social reinforcement and get rid of her supply of "irresistible" food. One successful experience, of course, does not guarantee another. She may very well resort to binge-ing at a later time or in another place. However, even if she does, a different sequence of events has taken place. If successful, she has eliminated binge-ing during a specific time interval (e.g., when she is on the job) or in a particular place (her car) or when she is with a certain person (her slim neighbor), something she had thought she could *never* do. In addition, by trying new strategies in these extremely difficult situations, the woman shows herself that she is capable of coping.

Lest she rehearse for tragedy or sabotage herself by choosing to remember past failures (with the built-in assumption that she will fail again), we ask her to *reward herself* for every success. For instance, if she is avoiding binge-ing at home, she should plan to do something she enjoys and can easily carry out. She might list five possibilities. For example, she might enjoy a hot tub, listen to her favorite record album, go to a movie or a play, or call someone to whom she truly enjoys talking. The list is endless once one begins to recognize how important it is to be nice to oneself *consistently* and at *appropriate* times. It is often helpful at this point in treatment to point to the irony of binge-ing and purging—though the binger is obsessed with her body, she does little to take care of it! In fact, she is well on the way to damaging her health. Thus, any new strategy should involve being "gentle" with herself, especially when she has genuinely been tried. With time and practice, many women are amazed at their progress.

What if the woman fails to keep to her goal contract and succumbs to a binge? Then she must be willing to try another strategy! But the bulimarexic is often quite myopic. She sees only one alternative to anxiety. After giving in to the binge, she immediately admits failure and compounds the error by grotesque gorging and purging. At a time when remaining rational and alert is absolutely crucial, she stops—surrendering to her emotions. In that moment, the battle is lost!

She should ask herself what her alternatives are now that she has made a mistake? There are always alternatives. One, the most common, is to purge and reinitiate the cycle. Another is to binge and then *stop and reevaluate* (troubleshoot) precisely what went wrong. In fact, unless she can make this reassessment, it is quite likely that a similar sequence of events will soon lead to further binges. If the woman cannot determine what "red lights" she raced through, she can always return to her first alternative—the purge. But, we ask her, what does she have to lose by reversing the sequence so that troubleshooting precedes purging or binge-ing yet again?

There is, however, still another alternative. She could binge and *reach out* for support. At this point in treatment, we ask everyone to consider the following problem: A woman who is doing quite well weeks after the termination of the group is telephoned by another group member who is in the midst of a binge. The former, for any number of reasons, feels incapable of supporting the latter. What would *you* do? The group discusses the problem without our help, pitting their new knowledge and clearly stated goals against the familiar attraction to being accommodating. This enables us—and the women—to see who needs further individualized work and in what areas such work will be necessary. For example, those who feel compelled to help despite their apparent inability or reluctance to get too involved need to understand better how important it is to be an honest partner. Those who recognize that they cannot be all things to all people (yet have difficulty accepting this) need to reexamine how the bionic woman syndrome sets them up for feelings of inadequacy and self-doubt. Those who decline to help someone in real distress, because they are "sure" that the person really does not need help, will need to learn to avoid interpretation and analysis. Those who, despite genuine understanding, realize that they cannot be with a friend for good reason are in touch with the major issues. What they do will typically be decided in the moment, as it must be when a bulimarexic is under stress.

What is particularly important, however, is how the woman feels *after* she has responded to the plea for help. There is, of course, no one right way to respond, and she may later feel she could have done better. But if she does not make the attempt, she fails to confront the old habits that have not served her well.

Finally, unless the bulimarexic is willing to take the risk of trying out new strategies, she is likely to remain locked into her behavior. During all those years of people-pleasing, bulimarexics appear to have forgotten or, in some cases, never really learned that psychological growth comes about through initiating change. Most of us, no matter how inhibited or conventional, struggle with two mutually incompatible desires. On the one hand, we crave predictability. It is easy to stay with the tried and true. We do not wish to appear the fool! On the other hand, we feel the need to change. How else can we feel accomplishment? If we are what we *do,* we must acknowledge that variety in our lives is a necessary precursor of psychological well-being. Although the consequences of risk taking certainly help to shape our lives, without the *process,* little learning can occur. With these thoughts in mind, what remains is to develop strategies based on well-conceived risks.

We have found it particularly helpful to remind our clients to pay careful attention to the "bottom line." We ask, what is the worst that could happen if you engage in a particular alternative? If the outcome is potentially devastating, the proposed strategy may be too extreme or in need of revision. For example, Sally had been living at home and working as a waitress for several months, having left college abruptly after a series of extreme binge / purge episodes. Bored and ashamed, she had been avoiding other people. Her parents, although supportive, felt compelled to lecture her about her future and what she should be doing. In the course of our group, Sally established the following strategy: She would quit her job, move out of her parents' home, find her own apartment, and enroll in a program in nutritional science at a state university.

Sally knows that she feels inadequate as a waitress, that her parents are right about what she should be doing, and that if she is to succeed, she must do something that satisfies her. So far so good. Now let us look at the bottom line: what if she does not like the university program or does not do well? In either case, she has learned a great deal more than she could have had she remained a discontented waitress. Furthermore, if she does not like it, she is at least in a better position to determine what parts of the entire process she did not enjoy. In this particular case, living alone proved to be a major stumbling block. After a semester of daily binge-ing at 4:00 P.M. when she was alone in her apartment, Sally took a further risk and found a roommate. She chose not to share her secret with this woman; however, they did agree to spend time together each afternoon studying. This was Sally's idea, proposed so that she could devote time to her studies at an hour of the day when she felt most vulnerable. The women studied together, and, under Sally's direction, both learned to reward themselves for their efforts by attending campus events, dating, and jogging. Soon, and for the first time, Sally was able to share her history with her roommate-friend. After that, she was able to laugh at the behavior she had so carefully concealed for six agonizing years. As she put it in a letter to us: "I now know that because I can laugh at binge-ing, I no longer fear it and can deal with it whenever I wish." Napoleon put it another way when he said that those who fear being conquered are already doomed!

Each of the women with whom we work enters therapy with a varying amount of "unfinished business." Several hours in the group are therefore devoted to troubleshooting those hurdles that are often considered insurmountable. In an attempt to convey how we approach this important work, we would like to present one group member's script:

Andrea's days are all pretty much the same. Her morning ritual begins with checking her stomach for signs of bloating and jumping on the scale for the bad news. She will weigh herself at least five times during the day. Agonizing over how she might stave off a binge, Andrea thinks ahead to lunch, vacillating between promising herself that she will fast the entire day and deciding to eat just yogurt. She deals with her children first, getting them fed, dressed, and off to school. Andrea enjoys the bickering and activity. Mornings are generally happy times. Binge-ing hasn't yet begun, and she vows that today will be different, although deep down she knows that it won't be.

After driving her four-year-old to preschool, she heads for the grocery store to replace the food she consumed yesterday. She chooses a different store each day because she is convinced that all the clerks know about her. Andrea buys food she knows the children will like, assuring herself that she is not going to eat such junk. For the rest of the morning, she involves herself with errands and volunteer activities in a frantic attempt to avoid being home, where binge-ing is easiest.

Having gotten through the morning without binge-ing, she collects her daughter from preschool and returns home to find beds unmade, laundry piled high, and breakfast dishes beckoning. Mildly hungry, Andrea decides to eat one cup of yogurt for lunch while fixing her daughter a sandwich. Hunger intensifies! She wants more! She sends her daughter outside to play. Aware that her house is a mess, that her friend is getting a new one, which she will decorate beautifully because she is so artistic and well organized, Andrea begins with the cookies.

Initially, eating seems pleasant. The first cookie tastes good, as does her child's leftover sandwich. She decides to make several more sandwiches while consuming the remainder of the cookies. Out of control, the binge becomes unpleasant, messy, and painful. Andrea then consumes copious amounts of water, milk, and juice as she has learned that vomiting is easier when she drinks a lot. In addition to the sandwiches and cookies, she eats a pound of cheese and a jar of peanut butter—all bought that morning to last the week. By now she feels about to explode!

She rushes to the bathroom. Cramming her finger down her throat and vomiting has become as habitual as struggling not to think about the waste of food, her lack of discipline, and her inordinate shame. Moments later Andrea scours the toilet, brushes her teeth, and weighs herself to be sure that none of the dreaded food is detectable. Returning to the kitchen, she calls her little girl so that they can make cookies. Her son will soon be home from school, and she has devoured all the snack food. As she beats the batter and licks her fingers, her second binge is initiated. The freshly baked bookies have dwindled from two dozen to eight by the time her son arrives. Andrea continues to binge, purging about an hour later. Realizing that her husband will soon be home and that she has consumed most of their intended dinner, she runs to the grocery store. Writing her second check of the day, she blames her husband, who she is certain desires her to be a petite, pretty housewife and mother.

Andrea returns home under pressure to prepare dinner. By now she has lost patience and is screaming and yelling at her family. Dinner takes place in an atmosphere of chaos. The kids are happy to have Dad home, so Andrea is left alone to clean up. As she does so, she continues to consume the leftovers. When she purges, she runs the water in the bathroom sink so no one will hear her retching. Vomiting is now quite painful; her throat is on fire, and the skin around her mouth is raw.

Her husband goes to bed at 10:00 P.M., suggesting that she do the same. Andrea feels too dirty and disgusting to make love and fails to understand how he could ever desire her, so she consumes a handful of laxatives to assure that all food will be removed. She watches TV for an hour, then joins her sleeping mate. At 3:00 A.M., as usual, she awakens feeling ravenous and ready to reinitiate the destructive cycle.

The past eight years have been a variation on this theme. Eating and obsessing about food have occupied an inordinate amount of Andrea's time. When she is not preoccupied with binge-ing, Andrea pores through countless books on nutrition, dieting, and the psychology of self-help. She has also developed a reputation as a gourmet cook and superb hostess.

All members of the group listened intently to Andrea's story and took notes at our insistence. We encouraged them to identify the specific behaviors that precipitated Andrea's binge-ing and purging and to help her troubleshoot these hurdles by concentrating on the way she chose to begin her day. Upon awakening, she immediately weighed herself, anticipating bad news. What purpose does this serve? If she recognizes this as a good example of rehearsing for tragedy, what alternatives does she have to call upon? At this point, Andrea was placed on the "hot seat." After considerable thought, she concluded that she did not have to weigh herself, indicating that she could instead go to her favorite room—the study—and begin to plan her day. Such an alternative was in no way unique. Andrea, as well as other group members, had used a similar strategy in situations of more obvious stress.

However, one alternative strategy, no matter how creative or exceptional, is seldom sufficient. The bulimarexic woman needs at least one further alternative as a back-up. The challenges of day to day living are rarely mastered with one strategy! Not only does evaluating alternatives stimulate thinking at a crucial time, it also serves as a bulwark against additional threat.

Another alternative involved getting rid of the bathroom scale. This was easy since Andrea was the sole observer of its daily bad news anyway. Knowing herself and her tendency to function best in structured situations, Andrea modified this alternative somewhat. Like many bulimarexics, she fondly spoke of the "good old days." At one time, she had been an avid tennis player, but had left the club because of her fear of food and disdain for those who idled away their lives around the courts. Getting rid of the scale and adding an early morning tennis match as a new activity therefore served as her second alternative. Her husband, Hal, played regularly, and she was still asked to play tennis by women friends whose company she used to enjoy. Furthermore, with the new indoor courts, foul weather could not serve as an excuse not to play.

Moving on, Andrea focused upon the volunteer work she had undertaken in hopes of avoiding binge-ing. Honest evaluation suggested that the volunteer work had created unlimited opportunities to binge. Since she never really enjoyed this work, she did it poorly, feeling guilty about her lack of interest. Other more dedicated and competent volunteers, who occasionally censured her, further compounded Andrea's guilt, which gave her a further incentive to engage in binge-ing. Upon reminding herself that a person is what he or she does, Andrea concluded that she had been an unfulfilled wife and mother in many regards. She therefore decided to set new goals. She would plan daily afternoon activities away from home with her daughter. Her son, Billy, could also be involved. After all, home had become her major setting for gorging and purging. At this point, a group member pointed out that someone had to make the bed, clean the house, and prepare the meals. Acknowledging this, Andrea again assumed responsibility. Aware that she was viewed as a woman of leisure because she had a master's degree and a lawyer husband who did not expect her to work, she felt that she should at least take care of her home. Nevertheless, she abhorred doing so. What were her alternatives? This time, Andrea quickly delineated three. First, she could do the work and then reward herself for having done so; along the way, she might also learn to accept strokes from others. Second, she could look for a part-time job and use some of the money to hire a maid. Finally, she could ask her children to help with the housework, thereby interacting with them in a more appropriate and rewarding way than she had before (i.e., as a model of cleanliness and discipline rather than as a person who is out of control and inconsistent) while teaching them how to clean and care for themselves and their surroundings.

Group members are usually excited and encouraged by the ease with which they help each other to generate alternatives. The process by which active strategies are arrived at is often contagious and may carry over to more realistic settings outside of the group. Evening homework assignments are designed to further elicit new responses to old situations. Because of the group's commitment to change, it soon becomes apparent that new habits can be substituted for old ones. What's more, as they pinpoint specific stimuli that bring on binge-ing, many women discover that what is necessary is a *relabeling* of the situation rather than a reliance upon new strategies. Labeling themselves as "aroused" or "excited" instead of as "hysterical" or "anxiety-ridden" allows them to *plan* rather than *retreat*.

After a few success experiences based on relabeling, most women see the benefits of this new way of responding. Troubleshooting strategies then may require further evaluation, but evaluation must now occur in an active realm. The women are likely to sabotage themselves if they try to think through each and every alternative, for we have found that bulimarexics can think themselves into or out of anything! This is the time for action. Whether various strategies can be easily integrated into daily life and whether relatives and friends will be sympathetic cannot be determined with certainty in advance. Each woman must therefore *react without expectation* once she has developed her alternatives. The worst that might happen is that she will not succeed. However, in the process, it is possible that she might discover, on her own or with the help of others, what led to a particular unsuccessful outcome.

Andrea had an experience that she spontaneously shared with the group. She felt that her sex life had been less than adequate ever since Hal and she had dated in college. She blamed this on bulimarexia. One night, in desperation, she decided to create a romantic setting in which to entertain Hal when he returned home that evening from a business trip. She sent the children to her mother's house for the night, dressed provocatively, chilled a bottle of wine, prepared an elegant meal, and awaited Hal's arrival by candlelight. When he arrived, he was overwhelmed by the reception. They made love magnificently, and Andrea remembered that evening for weeks thereafter. However, the pleasure of the occasion was not duplicated.

Andrea now revealed that it was primarily because of her expectations and lack of honest communication that she did not follow up on her sexual enjoyment with Hal. The problem was that she expected Hal to do something similar, and soon! After all, it was his turn, wasn't it? When he did not, she was sure it was because she was unattractive to him. Instead of communicating honestly with her husband, she assumed her interpretation was accurate and resumed her nightly binge-ing and purging. Hal's attempts to initiate further sexual involvement were thereby thwarted.

Realizing that she wanted a more fulfilling sexual experience with her husband, Andrea formulated new strategies. She decided to make a pact with herself. From now on she would *ask rather than interpret!* To begin with, she would attempt to initiate sexual encounters with Hal and encourage him to do so with her as well. Since she enjoyed being "social chairman," why not capitalize on this talent? In the next few months, Andrea found that she could effect significant changes in her sex life that carried over to married life in general. Much to her delight, Hal spent more time at home, and, with the help of a therapist, they began a new relationship based upon honesty and risk taking. Andrea occasionally overeats, but she no longer turns these infrequent lapses into extended binge / purge episodes. She has neither the time nor the inclination.

Although we had not originally intended it, our relationship as a couple often serves as a focal point for group discussion, since we tend to interact openly with one another. When we disagree before the group, our actions and words are often scrutinized in light of those crucial issues that are typically raised during the all-women session. Many of the fantasies and erroneous expectations that women attribute to men are thereby exposed. For example, most bulimarexics are convinced that men prefer to direct and teach women. Thus, when Marlene shows Bill where he is remiss, his response and her way of relating to him can be experienced directly. Quite spontaneously, we illustrate a variety of communicative skills that are foreign to many group members. In revealing our own struggles and deficiencies, we also help dispel the myth of the "perfect couple" and give the women another chance to evaluate and formulate new approaches to change. Therapists are not immune to maladaptive behavior and can also profit from the suggestions of the group. Thus, the group process has something to offer everyone.

BEHAVIOR REHEARSAL

The final phase of our treatment is devoted to leave-taking. By this time the women know how to deal with bulimarexia, but can they apply these new skills? In preparation for the challenges ahead, we ask each group member to articulate what she has learned. In effect, we facilitate a review of *the vocabulary of therapy*.

Throughout therapy we insist that the women take notes—jot down words, phrases, and concepts that serve as building blocks to a more productive life style. We point out that bulimarexia has consumed an inordinate amount of time and energy in the past that can now be devoted to *doing*—doing whatever *they* choose. Women have consistently written to tell us how valuable their notebooks were to them after the group. The following notes were shared with us by a former client, who, after eleven months of binge-free living, felt that her adherence to the following principles served to maintain her strides toward recovery.

Habit:	Bulimarexia is *not* a disease; it is a *learned* behavior that can be unlearned.
Responsibility:	Gorging and purging will continue unless the bulimarexic stops blaming other people and / or circumstances (i.e., "I flunked the exam because I binged" really means "I flunked it because I didn't study"). Take *responsibility* for the behavior.
Why:	Let go of the "whys" because you can never be sure if you are right. Ask instead: "What do I get from gorging and purging?" Then you will have some idea of what might replace these destructive behaviors.
Past / Present / Future:	"What tense am I in?" Give up dwelling on yesterday as well as rehearsing for tragedy in the future. Devote energy and attention to the *moment.* That's where you can make an impact.
Expectations:	Let go of expectations and begin *honest goal-contracting.* Expectations lead to disappointment, which fosters bulimarexia. Goals do not imply outcome, but represent a commitment to *trying.*
Pain:	Think of pain as a precursor to *change,* not to binge-ing. Learn from your

pain; and not how to avoid it. Don't court pain, but use it to motivate risk-taking. *Acting* rather than reacting is key to the process of change.

Risk-taking: Be willing to step into the unknown without being absolutely certain of the outcome. Progress is dependent upon trying new ways of living. If you don't like the outcome, you can go back to the way you were. Few things in life are irreversible.

Toxic words: Eliminate such words as *can't, forever,* and *never* from your vocabulary: they are steppingstones to *perfectionism* and to ultimate self-defeat. There are no bionic people!

Power: Don't give up your power by allowing others to control you. Don't say "yes" when you really mean "no." Take a careful look at your *audience.* Stop being a *people pleaser* and start making your *own* mistakes.

Mistakes: Nobody's perfect, so when you make a mistake stay in the here-and-now and troubleshoot. If you don't, you're likely to make the same mistake again and again.

Sabotage: Avoid those self-destructive yet tempting states of being (i.e., isolationism, perfectionism, pessimism, and inactivity). Identify your *rackets*— those behaviors that, in the long run, feed bulimarexia.

Ask: Don't interpret! With your self-concept, you're sure to expect the worst! Learn to ask rather than to analyze.

Identity: Oneness must precede twoness! Establish your identities. You are what you do. Self-respect is contingent upon success experiences. Learn to reinforce yourself so that growth is not based solely upon interactions with others. *Be kind to yourself in the face of stress* so that you can cope, rather than succumb to a binge. Enjoy your accomplishments. Practice giving as well as accepting strokes!

These important behavioral principles are the essence of treatment. Women who truly understand them usually make a commitment to change in unique ways. However, a new beginning in an old environment, often proves difficult. Furthermore, healthy strides need to be maintained *over time*. When they are not, it is fair to say that therapy has been of limited value. Thus, the final aspect of our treatment involves taking "psychological inventory." The time has come to determine whether the "well-educated" group member is now capable of handling the stressful situations that she is likely to encounter upon returning home.

CHAPTER 8

A Look to the Future

With each group the times comes when the work is nearly over and final leave-taking must take place. The women congratulate themselves and each other for the gains they have made, but they are apprehensive about returning home. The same old challenges and stresses will still be there, and the people who are important to them are not likely to have undergone any appreciable change. As a final exercise, we ask each woman to rehearse for tragedy—that is, to live in the future. By now, each one has a list of her salient "red lights"—the people, places, and attitudes that have invariably led to binge / purge behavior. In addition, each has delineated alternatives to binge-ing. Rehearsing for the future now represents an opportunity to apply new strategies to old situations. The woman can prove to herself that she is a different person in an important way.

This is a time of concerns and questions. Nearly every woman asks us: *When (and how) will I know I am no longer bulimarexic?* The question is natural considering the tenacity of the binge / purge syndrome; it represents the woman's fear that she can never be sure she is free of the

195

behavior. She is, of course, subscribing to the belief that serious habits, such as alcoholism, smoking, and drug abuse, must be eliminated completely if the outcome is to be successful. However, recent research into these problems has cast doubt on whether the all-or-nothing hypothesis is accurate. As far as bulimarexia is concerned, to insist that the bulimarexic can never take one mouthful of a forbidden food is simply unwarranted, as many women will attest. So the answer to the question of when and how bulimarexia becomes a behavior of the past depends on the individual and the goals she sets herself. For example, Laura, a former group member, writes: "It has been three years since the group, and I am now cured! Oh, I still overeat on occasion (about once a month) but I don't view it as the end of the world, and I don't use it as an excuse to engage in the old cyclic ritual. I now like my life *most* of the time, and, although I'm still lazy and find that I binge when I feel that way, I can deal with it because I own that part of me. It no longer owns me!"

Jill feels: "I'm not there yet! I have cut the frequency of my binges in half over the past year and haven't purged for over two years, but I still feel out of control when I resort to overeating. I've learned *a lot* but I want more therapy, so I have negotiated a new contract with my old therapist. We'll see how it goes."

Finally, Eve, who had been binge-ing and purging for eighteen years, had this to say thirty months after the group experience: "I'll never be completely happy unless I stop this forever. I know that this statement smacks of sabotage and just knowing that helps a great deal. It allows me to admit that I use eating as a way of avoiding intimacy. I still binge once in a while (once or twice a month), not out of habit, but in order to avoid men (at the same time, I continue to blame them for my loneliness). My purging is far less frequent now (six times last year), and my therapy is aimed much more at risk taking. I'm at peace with myself for the first time in years and am grateful for that. Perhaps I will stop this habit. However, if I don't, I can now get on with my life as I have been doing for the last two years. I will reach out to you again if I feel the need to stop permanently."

Thus, Laura is willing to believe that she is finished with bulimarexia, although she still overeats occasionally. She likes herself most of the time. She has given up certain absolutes and no longer believes that a lapse means she has failed; Laura knows that she does not have to be perfect and indeed will never be perfect.

Jill is more tentative, not willing to call herself "cured" because she still binges at times. But she is motivated enough to trust a therapist to help her cut down her need to binge and is hopeful. She knows she is not there yet, but has not dismissed the possibility that she can stop completely.

Eve admits to greater serenity, but knows she will not be satisfied until she stops completely. However, she is not ready to make a permanent commitment. This may be quite wise since, for the time being, she *knows* how she is using the behavior. When she is able to be more outgoing, more of a risk-taker, she will not have to fall back on bulimarexia.

The common denominator for all these women is, of course, their belief systems. Laura is confident, and Jill and Eve less so. Thus, despite comparable strides and strategies, these women respond to their success experiences and their failures differently.

These three women were at different stages of readiness

to give up bulimarexia. Two reached out for further therapy, often a good thing. A therapist who is knowledgeable about the problem, who does not judge and measure outcome by *his or her criteria,* may be able to speed the process of change. However, therapy is not a panacea for everyone struggling with bulimarexia. Many women are not ready to work on giving up binge-ing. Others are still looking for a magic solution. Still others are secretly looking for an excuse to continue, and these women seek therapy so they can claim they have "tried everything." As one woman candidly put it: "I wanted to be able to say, 'Well, I worked with the experts, but I'm still binge-ing.' " These women are, of course, covertly relying upon someone else to make everything right instead of tackling the problem themselves.

Fortunately, the majority of builmarexic women are intelligent. When therapy directly exposes their sabotage maneuvers, most will—at some time—try alternatives to binge-ing *on their own.* Women we have interviewed only once have called months later to tell us that they have been binge-free since they chose to initiate the call. The mere act of picking up the phone and calling us appeared to give them the strength they needed to begin to change. In effect, that phone call represented the first risk.

Recently, we have begun "booster treatment" programs with former clients to work on specific issues and unfinished business of the sort expressed by Jill and Eve. So far this format has proved to be an effective adjunct to our short-term group therapy program. The rewards are significant for us also since these programs enable us to keep in touch with many women we have come to know and respect. The following letter, addressed to the other members of a particular group, is illustrative:

"Dear Friends:

"I am writing to you to share some of my feelings and experiences since our weekend in Ithaca, and to tell you that I am celebrating over two years of freedom from bulimarexia! There have been some very tense, anxious moments, but I've gotten through them without resorting to my former way of coping with a good ole 'binge and purge' session. I am writing to say I care, and I hope that I can somehow send you some energy or strength, if you need it, to overcome this habit that we have lived with so long.

"I have decided to work with other women who, like us, are trying hard to free themselves of the behavior that we found so consuming. In talking with many women, I find I am most often asked what I have now replaced the behavior with. I wish I could say that another behavior fits the slot perfectly and relieves the inner tension as well. It simply isn't that easy. I think more than anything I have replaced binge-ing and purging with freedom, direction, and health. I look back on my seven years of bulimarexia as a sentence in which I was ruled, controlled, dominated, driven, and obsessed by a behavior that did not allow me to get on with my life, to accept responsibility for it, and quite frankly, to grow up! That is my freedom from the behavior, and I see my life moving in a direction in which I am leading and not being led as before.

"I have gotten through these past two years by taking them a day at a time. (There were some particularly difficult moments in which I focused on an hour at a time!) I have learned how to reach out when I feel weak and to allow others to help me by telling them what I need. I have called my husband and my sister when I was anxious or scared that binge-ing might reemerge and asked them for a shot of energy and strength to get back my resolve. I have kept myself from giving into the moment and blaming it on all those external forces. I have actually walked out of my house leaving behind the kitchen and other 'trigger places' to take a walk or a ride from the stimulus or set-up situations.

"Occasionally, I look back with sadness at having lost seven years of really productive living. Years when my priorities and focus were so out of line! I am ashamed of the abuse I put my body through, but I applaud my success! I have learned that it's nice to get strokes from others, but learning to stroke yourself is as important and as gratifying. I can still recreate the warmth of our weekend together in which we shared our strengths and weaknesses, where we learned that being helpless and weak had only fed our habits and made us dependent and victimized by our own design.

"I am still very concerned with being thin, but I am working hard on not putting all my energy into bodily perfection. I am trying to relax more, which is very hard for me, but a real goal yet to reach.

"I close with the hope that this letter finds you stronger and more determined in your efforts to be free of bulimarexia. I hope I have shared enough of myself to give you a sense of the happiness I have now found and the tremendous satisfaction that I feel at having beaten this habit. I would love to hear from you. I care, I'm with you, and I'm hoping that you are celebrating too!

> With my love,
> Rebecca"

Other questions women frequently ask are: *How will I deal with my parents, my husband, and my friends when I return home? How will I handle it when they ask, "What have you learned from therapy?"* It is natural for concerned loved ones to ask this question bluntly and directly. And it is natural for the bulimarexic woman, who hopes she will abandon the behavior entirely, to attempt to answer as directly and completely as possible. But though immediately asking the woman what she has learned may be legitimate, it can also be premature. How is the bulimarexic to know what she has learned until she has had a chance to apply her new knowledge and accumulate some successes? If she says, "I know I can quit," her expectations are probably unrealistic, at least at this time. One mistake and she is doomed. It would be much better if she answered in a more measured, provisional, and realistic way. Consider how nineteen-year-old Betsy answered the loaded question "What have you learned?" Her letter to us describes what she said to her parents:

"Well folks, I'm not sure. I have learned a lot about a part of me that I don't like anymore, but I also think I have consistently underestimated that part. I now think that I will need some help if I am to permanently overcome bulimarexia. I must do most of the work myself because I have chosen to binge. Drs. White will continue to support me and so will some of the women from the group, and I think I know how you can best help me. I may make some mistakes; so might you. If so, I want to learn from them so I don't keep making the same ones over and over again.

"I have not binged since I left the group and I feel strange physically. I want an appointment with our doctor. I want to be honest about the *whole thing* because I may have harmed myself by all of this. I also want to get back into my life as you have been urging me to. But Daddy, I don't like jogging, I just like the talks we have when we run. I don't want to give them up but I do want to get back into swimming and I wish you and Mom would join me. I am not happy with my job, so I'm going to look for another and will begin night school next month as we have so often discussed. I have no expectations but I want to use my savings to pay for the classes in order to motivate me to begin living again. This might also help me to stop binge-ing, since I usually do it between 6 and 9 P.M.

"I don't want to move out as I planned. I need your support. I need you to trust me again despite past deceit and disrespect. I intend to try to be honest because unless I do, I'll slow myself down for sure. I would like to try these things for six months and then see how I'm doing. Will you help me?"

Betsy's parents were willing to help, but skeptical. As it turned out, she was not binge-free during that six-month interval. However, she troubleshot her mistakes and, with the help of her parents, is now studying dental hygiene and has been binge-free for a year. Her life is filled with activities she enjoys, and she says: "I just don't have the time or the paralyzing inclination anymore!"

Betsy's clear statement about her immediate needs and goals was refreshing. She included rather than excluded her parents in her plans, with the result that they felt less anger and resentment toward her. Betsy's father wrote to us: "We are so pleased to have our daughter back. She left as an angry, frightened, unapproachable child and returned as a woman to be respected! We have played a small part in that metamorphosis and, as a result, feel like a family for the first time!"

Betsy's commitment represents an active pursuit of a

better lifestyle rather than a passive plea for attention. We were delighted but not surprised by the outcome.

We are often asked what parents, husbands, friends and lovers can do to help the bulimarexic recover. By now, it should be clear that very little of value can be done to or for the bulimarexic. Advice, recommendations, and threats only cause the woman to become more defiant of or dependent on those who are trying to help. Well-intentioned loved ones often set themselves up for a great deal of pain and frustration when they assume the role of caretaker. An exceptionally bright and competent attorney, the mother of one of our clients, decided that she was partially to blame for her daughter's behavior and became a "social policeman" by installing locks on kitchen cabinets for three weeks in order to "make it easier for Naomi to control herself." In so doing, the mother removed the temptation (food) and also monitored her daughter most evenings (with intermittent help from her silently begrudging husband). Naomi engaged in a variety of bizarre behaviors during this time, but did not binge. The mother felt sure that her daughter was, at long last, in control. Sanctions were lifted, and that same day Naomi engaged in her worst binge ever. The mother, shocked and disillusioned, sought professional help and was advised to hospitalize Naomi immediately. After two months in the psychiatric ward of a major metropolitan hospital, Naomi emerged angry, resentful, and feeling more hopeless than ever. Binge-ing and purging intensified. Family rapport was seriously jeopardized despite the fact that these three people had been fairly close one year earlier.

The bottom line for those who know or care about a bulimarexic is this: Do not take responsibility for her behavior by trying to fix her! If you fail, you and she both feel you are incompetent. If you succeed, the "victim" is dependent upon you. It is a no-win situation that is exceedingly difficult to resist, particularly for well-integrated, successful, caring people. The bulimarexic must initiate the process of change by herself making a commitment to doing something in her own behalf.

Over the past seven years, we have become painfully aware of the many ways that sex-role stereotyping has kept women from realizing their full potential. Our work has led us to strongly identify with women's struggles, and we have been outraged by the stories of misery, the reality of so many wasted lives and unfulfilled dreams. Witnessing such insidious societal pressures on our own children has reinforced our belief that today's parents and the parents of future female children must become more capable of guiding young women toward healthy independence as adults and must be determined to do so. Well-informed fathers must learn to encourage their daughters to achieve and compete instead of trying to protect them from challenge and responsibility. This is especially important in order to offset socialization pressures both within and outside the family. Recent studies of successful women have consistently revealed that they experienced unusually strong childhood relationships with fathers who encouraged risk taking, stamina, and strength of character rather than passivity and conventional femininity. Mothers also need to become more aware of the enormous power and impact they can have as models for their daughters. They must endeavor to broaden their activities in ways that engender self-respect and the respect of others. The parent who shows rather than tells offers an invaluable legacy.

However, this is not enough. On radio and television, in magazine advertisements and films, we are constantly bombarded with unrealistic and unhealthy models of womanhood. As a result, hundreds of thousands of young women strive for a feminine ideal that is practically impossible to attain. The ramifications are horrifying, especially in terms of the major health threat we are presently witnessing. Who is deciding how slim women should be and what they should look like? Responsibility rests with all of us to demand healthier models, well developed and fit, to replace the weak and emaciated ones whose very presence conveys the destructive, subliminal message—"If you could lose five more pounds you would be perfect."

Women need to recognize their power as consumers. They can lobby and boycott products that reiterate and exploit these distorted ideals. Models and actresses who are forced by the merchandising and entertainment establishments to achieve unhealthily slim bodies could attempt to resist these pressures in concerted and united ways. In the past, groups of women have banded together admirably and effectively. Airline stewardesses successfully defended efforts to discriminate against them in terms of age and marital status.

In this same vein, coaches of dance and athletics must become more aware of their influence. They need to become more informed about the physiological and psychological ramifications of eating disorders; they also would be well advised to study nutrition. Only then will they recognize the potential damage caused by distorted and unrealistic perceptions about body weight. For example, the historical ritual of "weighing in" in front of an audience can create extreme anxiety. The sensitive coach might recommend that an "overweight" child see a nutritionist or physician who could help to support and educate her in her attempts at weight regulation. At the same time, the ill effects that dieting can have on performance and stamina need to be emphasized. Finally, the youngster should not be given ultimatums with regard to weight loss lest she resort to strategies like bulimarexia.

School systems, colleges, and universities have the power and the means to offset some of the more crippling effects of these prevalent "antifat attitudes." Health education courses could routinely provide relevant reading material, guest speakers, and forums for interaction that might serve to curtail and ultimately prevent the epidemic of eating disorders sweeping the United States today. For example, females in elementary schools and in junior and senior high schools, who represent a "high-risk" population, might be screened using a body cathexis test and questionnaire. Those who loathed their bodies could then be invited to participate in "rap groups" with trained psychologists, nutritionists, and nurses in order to explore their feelings and discover more appropriate, healthy, and realistic ways of achieving goals. Such pilot programs are now being undertaken at Cornell. So far the results are encouraging. In the final analysis, preventive strategies will prove much more useful than curative efforts.

Recently, public awareness of eating disorders has increased significantly. Anorexia aid societies throughout the country have provided an effective means of support for desperate women, their parents, and other loved ones. Many of these organizations offer weekly group therapy programs and lecture series for anorexics, bulimarexics, and their families.

Self-help groups have also been organized for women with eating disorders. Cross-country networks have been established, often with the guidance and leadership of women who once struggled with *and overcame* these same problems. These women who have succeeded are role models for others; they share invaluable insights and offer concrete suggestions stemming from their own tribulations and successes. Through these kinds of supportive consciousness-raising experiences, women gain a more balanced perspective not only about their own bodies, but about the stifling aspects of the role assigned to them by society.

Women who are interested in joining a self-help group— or in forming one—should write to an anorexia aid society in their area. We are not able to list all of these organizations, but can suggest a few that cover most geographical areas of the United States. These organizations, in turn, can give you more specific advice.

For help in the West write to:

Anorexia Nervosa & Related Eating Disorders, Inc. (ANRED)
Post Office Box 5102
Eugene, Oregon 97405

In the Midwest:

Anorexia Nervosa and Associated Disorders, Inc. (ANAD)
Post Office Box 271
Highland Park, Illinois 60035

National Anorexic Aid Society, Inc. (NAAS)
Post Office Box 29461
Columbus, Ohio 43229

In the East and New England:

American Anorexia Nervosa Association, Inc. (AANA)
133 Cedar Lane
Teaneck, New Jersey 07666

The Anorexia Nervosa Aid Society of Massachusetts, Inc. (ANAS)
P. O. Box 213
Lincoln Center, Massachusetts 01773

In the South:

Maryland Association for Anorexia Nervosa and Bulimia, Inc.
(MAANA)
222 Gateswood Road
Lutherville, Maryland 21093

There are other self-help possibilities to consider. Overeaters Anonymous has been cited frequently by our clients as being exceedingly helpful. Women's consciousness-raising groups are also helpful, as are assertiveness training courses. While these suggestions should not be thought of as substitutes for a well-conceived therapy, if women are motivated to change their behavior, the prognosis is good. Women can also consult an endocrinologist or nutritional counselor or their own internists. These practitioners will be able to assess current health status and to discuss ways of combating physiological damage that may have resulted from bulimarexia, while at the same time offering preventive strategies.

For women who seek therapy, it would be wise to ask questions about the approach and philosophy of the therapist during an initial exploratory session. For instance, will the therapy focus on the present habitual response, with strategies for eliminating the binge / purge behavior, or will it concentrate on past, underlying conflicts? Does the therapist advocate a long- or short-term treatment? Will the sessions be individual or utilize a group approach? Has the therapist been successful in treating bulimarexia?

Once therapy is underway, progress should be evident

in several weeks. If not, both client and therapist should reexamine mutual goals in order to establish the most effective strategies or to ascertain whether the particular therapist / client relationship should be continued.

For help in finding a knowledgeable and reputable therapist in a particular region of the United States, women may write to the authors at *67 West Malloryville Road, Freeville, New York 13068.* Please enclose a stamped, self-addressed envelope. We will answer all inquiries and supply a reading list of material about bulimarexia.

In the meantime, here is a list of selected books and articles that may prove helpful:

1. BOOKS:

Beller, Anne S. *Fat and Thin: A Natural History of Obesity.* New York: McGraw-Hill, 1977.
Berne, Eric. *Games People Play.* New York: Ballantine, 1978.
Chernin, Kim. *The Obsession: Reflections on the Tyranny of Slenderness.* New York: Harper & Row, 1981.
Chesler, Phyllis. *Women and Madness.* New York: Avon Books, 1973.
Dowling, Collette. *The Cinderella Complex: Women's Hidden Fear of Independence.* New York: Summit Books, 1981.
Ehrenreich, Barbara and English, Deirdre. *For Her Own Good: 150 Years of the Experts' Advice to Women.* New York: Anchor Books, 1979.
Friedan, Betty. *The Feminine Mystique.* New York: W. W. Norton and Company, 1963; 2nd ed., 1974; paper, New York: Dell, 1977.
—. *It Changed My Life: Writings on the Women's Movement.* New York: Random House, 1976.
Hall, Lindsey, with Cohn, Leigh. *Eat Without Fear.* Santa Barbara, Calif.: Gurze Books, P.O. Box 20066, Santa Barbara, CA 93120. (This is the short story of a self-cured bulimarexic.)
Harris, Thomas. *I'm OK, You're Ok.* New York: Harper & Row, 1969; paper, New York: Avon Books, 1973.
Hawkins, R. C. II, Fremouw, W. J., and Clement, P. F., eds.: *Binge Eating: Theory, Research and Treatment.* New York: Springer Publishing Company. In press.

Liu, Aimee. *Solitaire.* New York: Harper & Row, 1979; paper, Harper & Row, 1980.

Lurie, Alison. *The Language of Clothes.* New York: Random House, 1981.

Orbach, Susie. *Fat Is a Feminist Issue.* New York: Paddington Press, 1978; paper, New York: Berkley Books, 1979.

Peele, Stanton and Brodsky, Archie. *Love and Addiction.* New York: Taplinger Publishing Company, 1975; paper, New York: New American Library, 1976.

Rivers, Caryl, Barnett, Rosalind, and Baruch, Grace. *Beyond Sugar and Spice: How Women Grow, Learn, and Thrive.* New York: G. P. Putnam's Sons, 1979; paper, New York, Ballantine, 1981.

Russianoff, Penelope. *Why Do I Think I Am Nothing Without a Man?* New York: Bantam Books, 1982.

Vincent, L. M. *Competing with the Sylph: Dancers and the Pursuit of the Ideal Body Form.* New York: Andrews & McMeel, 1980; paper, New York: Berkley Books, 1981.

Weideger, Paula. *Menstruation and Menopause: The Physiology and Psychology, the Myth and the Reality.* New York: Alfred A. Knopf, 1976.

2.   ARTICLES:

Boskind-Lodahl, Marlene. "Cinderella's Stepsisters: A Feminist Perspective on Anoerxia Nervosa and Bulimia." *Psychology of Women: Selected Readings,* ed. Juanita H. Williams, W. W. Norton and Company, 1979. Pp. 436–48. (Published originally in *Signs: The Journal of Women in Culture and Society,* vol. 2, no. 2, Winter 1976, pp. 342–56.)

Boskind-Lodahl, Marlene and Sirlin, Joyce. "The Gorging-Purging Syndrome." *Psychology Today,* March 1977, pp. 50–52.

Brenner, Marie. "Bulimarexia." *Savvy: The Magazine for Executive Women,* June 1980, pp. 54–59.

White, William C. and Boskind-White, Marlene. "An Experiential-Behavioral Approach to the Treatment of Bulimarexia." *Psychotherapy: Theory, Research and Practice,* vol. 18, no. 4, Winter 1981, pp. 501–507.

Young, Nancy. "Full Stomachs/Empty Lives." *Glamour,* September 1979, pp. 204–206. (Also see editorial in the December 1979 issue of *Glamour* about the response to the September article.)

Index